Routledge Revivals

Self-Care

Drawing on the concepts and resources developed at the first international symposium on the role of the individual in primary care, the authors of this book, originally published in 1977, delineate self-care and its relationship to professional care, reasons for the interest in self-care and a framework for future research. Self-care is a major factor in health and holds promise of even greater impact through educational development, the authors argue. They maintain that self-care is additive to society's ability to overcome many existing barriers to health care accessibility, quality and accountability. In this sense, the authors argue, self-care must be viewed as the first option, with any alternatives involving professional care gives being supportive and residual.

This volume played an important role in the research on self-care which surged during the 1970s.

Self-Care

Lay Initiatives in Health

Lowell S. Levin, Alfred H. Katz and Erik Holst

Routledge
Taylor & Francis Group

First published in Great Britain in 1977 by Croom Helm Ltd

This edition first published in 2026 by Routledge
4 Park Square, Milton Park, Abingdon, Oxon, OX14 4RN

and by Routledge
605 Third Avenue, New York, NY 10158

Routledge is an imprint of the Taylor & Francis Group, an informa business

ISBN: 978-1-041-34840-5 (hbk)
ISBN: 978-1-003-79480-6 (ebk)
ISBN: 978-1-041-34851-1 (pbk)

Book DOI 10.4324/9781003794806

SELF-CARE
Lay Initiatives in Health

Lowell S. Levin, Alfred H. Katz,
Erik Holst

CROOM HELM LONDON

First published in Great Britain 1977

Croom Helm Ltd, 2–10 St John's Road, London SW11

ISBN 0–85664–570–2

Printed in Great Britain by Biddles Ltd, Guildford, Surrey

CONTENTS

Acknowledgments

This book is the direct outgrowth of the International Symposium on The Role of the Individual in Primary Health Care, held in Copenhagen, Denmark, August 11–15, 1975. The contribution of Symposium participants must be acknowledged as the prime resource and reference for many of the ideas and issues which are elaborated in this document. It would be difficult to overstate the productivity of their deliberations, the creative and incisive insights they shared, and their reasoned argumentation on issues and needed research. Although it is not feasible to sort out individual contributions in this group effort, it is important to emphasize our appreciation for the helpful background and contributed papers by John Fry, Henry Lennard, Poul Pedersen, Lois Pratt, Keith Sehnert, and C. Harvey Smith. We also acknowledge with thanks the contributions of graduate students at the Yale University Department of Epidemiology and Public Health to the annotated bibliography on self-care.

Planning an international conference is always an arduous task. The usual complexities are compounded when the meeting objective is to break new conceptual ground and stimulate or redirect scholarly interest in it. So much depends on the selection of participants and the design and management of the meeting to take best advantage of their presence. This responsibility was undertaken by a planning committee co-chaired by Erik Holst and Marsden Wagner. Its membership included Paul Backer, Alfred Katz, Lowell Levin, Philip Selby, and R. Glyn Thomas.

We are indebted to E. Maurice Backett, Rapporteur for the Symposium, whose thoughtful and balanced summary greatly assisted the authors in the task entrusted to them. Indeed, the approach adopted for this book was in response to his recommendation that the Symposium Report be substantive beyond the literal proceedings.

An excellent technical staff backed up the work of the planning group and made the wheels turn. Our special appreciation is offered to Janine Morgall and Rose Marie Vergo as the Symposium secretariat; to Karen Gordon and Ron Somers who assisted as recorders; to Elisabeth Lorenzi who tied up the loose ends related to editorial organization; to Marcia Richardson for editing and proofreading;

and to Margaret Gibbs and Cynthia Goldblatt who typed the manuscript of this book.

The authors are indebted especially to the University of Copenhagen/University of California (UCLA) Joint Center for Studies of Health Programs which, in collaboration with the Sandoz Institute for Health and Socio-Economic Studies, Geneva, organized the Symposium; and to the Danish Medical Research Council which gave generous financial assistance to the Symposium. The Symposium discussions were greatly facilitated by the excellent meeting accommodations of the European Regional Office of the World Health Organization.

Symposium Participants

Paul Backer, M.D.
Professor of General Medicine, Institute of General Medicine, University of Copenhagen, Copenhagen, Denmark

E. Maurice Backett, M.B., B.S., F.R.C.P., D.P.H.
Professor and Chairman, Department of Community Health, University of Nottingham Medical School, Nottingham, England

Niels Bentzen, M.D.
Hospital Doctor, Department of Pediatrics, Odense University Hospital, Odense, Denmark

Craig D. Burrell, M.D.
Vice President, External Affairs, Sandoz, Inc., East Hanover, New Jersey, U.S.A.

Karl Evang, M.D.
Consultant, Norwegian Ministry of Social Affairs; Member, World Health Organization Panel on Health Administration, Oslo, Norway

Jørgen Fog, M.D.
Department Head, Primary Health Care and Medical Education, National Health Service of Denmark, Copenhagen, Denmark

Howard E. Freeman, PH.D.
Professor and Director, Institute for Social Science Research, University of California, Los Angeles, California, U.S.A.

John Fry, M.D., F.R.C.S., F.R.C.G.P.
General Practitioner, Beckenham, Kent, England

Victor R. Fuchs, PH.D.
Professor and Vice President—Research, National Bureau of Economic Research, Stanford, California, U.S.A.

Bernard Gampel, M.B.CL.B., D.P.H.
Head, Family Medicine Unit, Department of Social Medicine, Hebrew University—Hadassah Medical School, Jerusalem, Israel

Erik Holst, M.D.
Chairman and Co-director, U.C.L.A.–University of Copenhagen Joint Center for Studies of Health Programs, Institute of Social Medicine, University of Copenhagen, Copenhagen, Denmark

Svend Juul, M.D.
Assistant Professor, Institute of Social Medicine, Aarhus University, Aarhus, Denmark

Finn Kamper-Jørgensen
Member, Danish Medical Research Council and Senior Research Fellow, Institute of Social Medicine, University of Copenhagen, Copenhagen, Denmark

Alfred H. Katz, M.A., D.S.W.
Professor, School of Public Health, Center for the Health Sciences, University of California, Los Angeles, California, U.S.A.

Henry L. Lennard, B.S., PH.D.
Professor and Director, Family Study Section, University of California, San Francisco, California, U.S.A.

Lowell S. Levin, ED.D., M.P.H.
Associate Professor, Department of Epidemiology and Public Health, Yale University School of Medicine, New Haven, Connecticut, U.S.A.

Charles E. Lewis, M.D., SC.D.
Professor and Head, Division of General Internal Medicine and Health Services Research, Department of Medicine, University of California, Los Angeles, California, U.S.A.

Mary Ann Lewis, B.S., M.S.
Program Director, University of California Primex Program, Los Angeles, California, U.S.A.

Carl Erik Mabeck, M.D.
General Practitioner, Copenhagen, Denmark

Carlos J. Martini, M.D., D.P.H., M.P.H., M.SC., M.F.C.M.
Deputy Director, Health Services Research Group, Department of Community Health, University of Nottingham Medical School, Nottingham, England

Poul Axel Pedersen, M.D.
Chairman, Research Council and College of General Practitioners, Copenhagen, Denmark

Lois Pratt, PH.D.
Professor, Department of Sociology, Jersey City State College, Jersey City, New Jersey, U.S.A.

Julius A. Roth, PH.D.
Professor, Department of Sociology, University of California, Davis, California, U.S.A.

Keith W. Sehnert, M.D.
Director, Center for Continuing Health Education, Georgetown University, Arlington, Virginia, U.S.A.

Philip Selby, B.A., M.B., B.CHIR.
Sandoz Institute for Health and Socio-Economic Studies, Geneva, Switzerland

C. Harvey Smith, M.P.H.
Director, Health Education, Group Health Cooperative of Puget Sound, Seattle, Washington, U.S.A.

Marsden G. Wagner, M.D., M.P.H.
Associate Clinical Professor, University of California, Los Angeles, California, U.S.A.; and Co-director, U.C.L.A.–University of Copenhagen Joint Center for Studies of Health Programs, University of Copenhagen, Copenhagen, Denmark

John David Williamson, M.B.
Lecturer, Department of General Practice, Guy's Hospital Medical School, London, England

Herbert F.K. Zöllner, PH.D.
Health Planning and Evaluation Officer, World Health Organization, Regional Office for Europe, Copenhagen, Denmark

CHAPTER I

Introduction and Background

In August 1975, twenty-nine scholars from four European countries, Israel, and the United States met in Copenhagen at what appears to have been the first international symposium to give particular and exclusive attention to the role of individuals and families in the primary health care process. This gathering of social scientists, physicians, health administrators, and educators undertook a pioneering effort (1) to explore the concept of the lay contribution in primary health care; (2) to clarify assumptions of role and function; (3) to draw attention to relevant technical and social issues; and (4) to identify priority research needs.

The impetus for the Symposium was clearly part of a rapidly growing world interest in improving the quality, availability, and accessibility of primary health care resources as the keystone in medical care. Recent years have seen a plethora of approaches to the issues of primary health care delivery, directed at one or another aspect of this complex problem. We have seen efforts to correct imbalances in the deployment of primary medical personnel through incentive programs or other devices to encourage (and in some instances, compel) physicians and others to practice in underserved areas, especially in rural areas and among the urban poor. Short of instances where there have been major revisions in the political and social structure of the society,[1] re-deployment efforts have, on the whole, been disappointing.

We have seen, too, innovations in health care organization which were intended to enhance the efficiency of the primary health resource. Here the problem often has been one of overcoming inertia within the care system and "self-interested resistance."[2] Theory has been difficult to translate into practice, although there are again important exceptions in the case of national health services, family care teams, community health centers, and other manipulations of the professional resource.

There also has been an impressive range of efforts to meet the primary health care needs by revising the focus and methods of professional education in health, particularly that of physicians. The goal has been more emphasis on preventive medicine, community health, and family practice, with a variety of attractive options so students can experience primary care practice at first hand from social and personal as well as technical perspectives. Again, with some outstanding exceptions, the great majority of medical students, for well-known reasons, are still attracted to specializations, or to practice opportunities which (1) are highly dependent on elaborate and expensive technology; and (2) are situated in milieux rich in academic and social amenities.

Such efforts to strengthen and expand the professional resource in primary care will undoubtedly continue, especially undertakings which emphasize teamwork and the use of new health professionals. The concept of the physician extender, for example, will probably continue to proliferate and mutate through experience. But even these solutions to increasing the effectiveness of primary health manpower resources have their own limits—some having to do with legal and technical affiliation with the physician or an institution; others having to do with increasing costs of an already very expensive social institution. We are reminded by economists that health care is labor-intensive and that solutions to health care needs must be found which are socially responsible and economically tolerable. The pertinent question is: Do realistic solutions to primary health needs (in medical, social, and economic terms) lie totally or largely within the domain of the current and projected professional health manpower resources?

Professor Victor Fuchs responds in this way:

> By changing institutions and creating new programs we can make medical care more accessible and deliver it more efficiently, but the greatest potential for improving health lies in what we do and don't do for and to ourselves. The choice is ours.[3]

Similar conclusions were drawn by conferees at another international symposium on "The Limits of Medicine" held in Switzerland in March 1975. In closing that conference, Doctor Alex Comfort observed:

> If we look at medicine in general, I think it has already trended away from its past commodity and technology image by the logic of its research future. Some of its most promising innovations in medical technique already involve active patient self-help in a social setting—group therapy, the psychotherapeutic community and social learning experiences such as assertion training in psychiatry; biofeedback and operant conditioning for the control of automatic processes in the field of therapeutics. This, if we can develop it, promises a technology of

> medical self-control which has the potential for substituting almost wholly for drugs, in the management of conditions such as epilepsy . . . hypertension and anxiety . . .[4]

Our experience, our commitment to professional intervention in health, even our research and planning orientation in health have been based on the heretofore unchallenged assumption that the professional, or professionally controlled, resource is the universal and exclusive resource in health care. We have neglected or have been unaware, or perhaps have avoided consideration, of the individual and family as a present and potential source of health expertise. There are, of course, some exceptions to this—for example, in the care of diabetes and, more recently, hypertension. But, by and large, our concentration has been on recruiting people into society's health care machinery, under the designated competent authority of physicians. At best, we appear to have lacked confidence or trust in the lay resource; and at the most negative extreme have denigrated lay involvement in self-care as misinformed and dangerous, the result of "rampant empiricism."[5]

The Copenhagen discussions were not inhibited by such presumptions of professional exclusiveness in health care, or by belief in the inherent incapacity of the layperson to develop as an effective health resource in primary care. On the contrary, the Symposium was planned with the view that a viable preventive and therapeutic partnership between individuals, patients, and families and the professional health care worker is not only desirable but may be essential to achieve improved access, enhanced quality of care, better accountability, and lower costs. This was, in effect, the working hypothesis for the Symposium and formed the basis for its agenda.

The Symposium's first goal was to clarify the assumptions upon which the role of laypersons and families in primary care are presently approached. What do we assume, for example, to be the prerogatives of individuals and families in primary health care, both from the standpoints of current technical capability (child rearing, disease prevention, illness management) and from the standpoint of human and political rights to self-protection and participation in health care decision-making? What are the assumptions about the relationship of medicine to society—the nature of the unwritten social contract between providers and clients—and medicine's potential for changing or reducing the degree of professional control in health care?

In preparation for the Symposium, a scan of the literature on the role of individuals and families in primary care revealed a burgeoning public interest and complementary political rationales. We found a few purposeful education programs which were actually in operation, particularly in the United States, and aimed at strengthening lay health care skills. We were also struck by an extraordinary array of instructional guides and protocols designed to enhance laypersons' functioning in primary health care.

Overall, the impression was gained from the literature of a spontaneous popular phenomenon, as yet little influenced by technical research inputs from behavioral scientists and clinicians. Furthermore, the literature review produced little evidence of evaluative research and this was mostly fragmentary, limited in scope, unrelated to a conceptual framework, or flimsy in design. Almost totally absent was research addressed to the transcending issues of lay participation in health care: e.g., the lay and professional barriers that inhibit role revisions; the technical, legal, economic, and educational processes required for the functional transfer of health care knowledge and skills from professionals to the laity; and the thorny questions of quality control. If, as some believe, a new lay-professional partnership may emerge, then there is a clear and pressing need for studies of its impact on cultural, economic, personnel, and other policy questions.

The Symposium sought to look squarely at the present phenomena that are broadly grouped under the rubric of self-care. It strove to elucidate the potential role of laypersons in primary health care in terms that could provide a framework for cooperative international efforts and cross-cultural studies; that could test the efficacy of culturally and socially specific approaches to lay education in primary care; and that could monitor or evaluate the effects of self-care in health. The last point was given special emphasis. It became clear in discussion that one need is for evaluative strategies that go beyond the usual measurements of the benefits of health care, i.e., absence of disease or treatment outcomes. When health care initiatives are shared by laypersons and professionals, changes can be anticipated in the health decision-making process, in the phenomenon associated with patient dependence, and in iatrogenic effects. Given a broad perspective on the health care system as encompassing the total social resource, measurements of outcomes need to be expanded to include a commensurately broad range of variables that reflect the general public welfare. This also will require observation of changes in normative factors not usually considered in health services evaluation, e.g., concepts of deviance and levels of functional autonomy in health care.

The decision to focus the Symposium on the role of the layperson as a self-provider of primary health care was not intended as a blind faith gesture in support of or in opposition to this role. Yet the very process of recognizing the existence of self-care as a major factor in primary health care, and of raising questions concerning its contributions and potentials raised concern that objectivity might give way to "evangelism." And there was no doubt that the issue of lay initiatives in primary care evoked strong personal and professional values, often expressed in statements of belief rather than fact. Limited time did not allow sufficient opportunity for adequate exploration, challenge, rebuttal, and synthesis, but the major issues and research needs were sharply etched and are reported in this book.

The work of the Symposium was concentrated in three groups meeting concurrently. Membership in each group was determined largely on the basis of disciplinary preference and experience. An effort also was made to achieve a good international balance. The working groups' agendas were planned around three topics, with the role of the individual and family as the general reference point: (1) economics, social planning, and administrative practice; (2) health and educational practice; and (3) social and behavioral sciences. An agenda placed before each group suggested modes for discussion, but was not expected to be adhered to strictly. The intent was to establish a frame of reference for each group which could help assure coverage of major aspects while minimizing intra- and inter-group redundancy. Brief summaries of group deliberations were presented to the Symposium, each forming the subject of a plenary session. Discussions throughout were extraordinarily rich, as evidenced in the unabridged form of the taped transcript. There was nuance, there were idea fragments, and that level of meaning which is inherent in the juxtaposition of intense discourse. On the other hand, fifty hours of recorded discussion disclosed a good amount of discursive and repetitive material which only occasionally followed sustained and full argumentation. Background concepts relevant to self-care were often referred to but rarely discussed in detail. At this stage in the development of our understanding of self-care as a factor in primary health care it was decided to avoid, where possible, theoretical excursions in favor of gaining some overall picture. On balance, this appears to have been a correct strategy as measured in the yield of central policy and research issues proposed. But there is no doubt that the inability to elaborate basic theoretical parameters (e.g., belief model, decision theory) diminished some opportunities for consensus and occasionally obscured the basis of dissent.

The following chapters present an overview of self-care, its function in primary care, some of the main issues that arise in considering its future development, and the challenges it poses in research. Rather than undertaking a literal precis of the Symposium discussions, the authors have drawn heavily from them, but have supplemented them, weaving back and forth in order to present a more coherent perspective. This process of selection was necessarily judgmental in the interests of culling the major ideas and issues that would stimulate scholarly and lay interest in self-care. It is necessarily a tentative and unfinished work, a review of the state of our knowledge of self-care and of the many questions which arise about its status and potential in meeting primary health care needs. Many issues raised could not be handled here.

It should be noted that this book is interpretive and elaborative rather than reportorial in character. The authors were stimulated and guided by perspectives and ideas generated by the Copenhagen Symposium, but were not constrained by them. We accept full responsibility for the text and any error of fact or fault of interpretation. No attempt was made to seek the endorsement or appraisal of this text by either participants or sponsors, and no such endorsement is implied or should be assumed.

References

[1]Joshua Horn, *Away With All Pests* (New York and London: Monthly Review Press, 1969).

[2]Irving K. Zola and John B. McKinley, *Organizational Issues in the Delivery of Health Services* (New York: Prodist, 1974).

[3]Victor R. Fuchs, *Who Shall Live?* (New York: Basic Books, 1974), p. 151.

[4]Alex Comfort, remarks recorded at the International Symposium "The Limits of Medicine," held March 24–26, 1975, in Davos, Switzerland (Gottlieb Duttweiler-Institute, Rüschlikon-Zurich).

[5]National Analysts, Incorporated, *A Study of Health Practices and Opinions* (Springfield, Virginia: National Technical Information Service, U.S. Department of Commerce, June 1972), pp. 15–16.

CHAPTER II

Self-Care in Health Care

The Social Nature of Self-Care

People are not accustomed to thinking about living in technical terms, even though breakdowns in the living process are often described as failures to cope effectively in biological, psycho-social, or economic spheres. People do not have explicit awareness of living as a complex of technologies, conventional wisdom, and rules of conduct. Indeed it has sometimes taken the objectifying effect of parody to reveal the nature of our ordinary life technology.[1] This is especially the case when it comes to aspects of living which are not dramatic departures from the routines of behavior. These are the ordinary things we do in ordinary ways, which are noticed or acknowledged only in their absence. A host of body rituals like brushing teeth and bathing are examples. These are not undertaken lightly, nor do they lack technology, cognate and belief material, or planning and evaluation. But they are culturally fused behaviors, for the most part universal, routine, self-initiated, self-maintained, and self-monitored. Socialization of the child, together with some supplementary formal training, contributes a myriad of living (self-caring, self-preserving) behaviors which are taken for granted as a sort of baseline of responsible human activities, contributing to an individual's or group's competence. Indeed, the categorization of such self-care competencies forms a good part of the anthropological grid for cultural analysis and comparison.[2]

Some categories of coping behavior, including those behaviors described as health behavior, appear to be more amenable to identification and typing than others. Perhaps this is a function of their observability, but, more probably, the ease of identification of coping behavior has to do with the degree to which meaning must be inferred from observed behavior. An act of preparing food as a prelude to eating may be described with little dispute about the observed facts. To label food preparation as health behavior, however, as involving nutritional decisions on the part of the cook, may be more hazardous. On the other hand, no life practices can be absolutely ruled out as health practices. Criteria to determine such a judgment are complex. The argument that distinctions can be made between behaviors which influence health and those which are purposeful health behaviors may be convenient, but, given the pervasive and diffuse nature of health, it offers little more than insight into the biases of the observer.

An holistic approach to health behavior cautions that it is essential to broaden our perspective on health behaviors beyond those which have become professionally legitimated. The holistic orientation assumes that health is an attribute of individual and group behavior; its integrity is heightened by its pervasiveness rather than its divisibility. The panoply of health behaviors should be accepted and acknowledged without regard to their technical fit into criteria or categories derived solely from a professional rather than a popular base. At the moment, we need assume nothing with regard to the efficacy of those behaviors. We need only agree that health behavior is a cultural idea. Cultural factors define its benefits as well as its distribution. The isolation of specialized health behaviors as contributing to well-being (cf. the World Health Organization definition of health) is difficult to achieve in any universal way, given the highly relative notion of health itself. A strategy for describing individual health behavior inevitably derives from an individual's or group's self-observations, insights, and motivation to share these data with others. The availability of professional technology to facilitate this process is still in question. As John Williamson observes, one challenge to the health professions is ". . . to step outside of a medical model of the health/disease issue and to take into consideration the value components of healthward care as perceived by the actors themselves."[3] The implied revisions in both professional perspectives and research technologies in health are discussed in Chapter IV.

Coping with disease or injury, once it has occurred, is more easily identified as discrete behavior. Deviance, by definition, calls attention to itself and makes its own demands on individuals and groups for response, be it to reduce the lesion or to undertake socio-psychological accommodation. And although "deviance" is itself a culturally determined concept, coping and preventive behavior designed to forestall further problems is usually concrete and measurable both in its effectiveness and extent. A vast research literature on public knowledge, attitudes, and behavior relating to specific diseases or injuries is available, but most of these studies are geared to contributing a data base for professional health interventions.[4] Professionals' concerns about what the public is doing about health mainly revolve around popular recognition of the need (1) to accept professional advice regarding health promotion or disease prevention; and (2) to enter the professional health care system for prophylaxis, diagnosis, or treatment. This bias in the research clearly reflects more general social values of the salience of professional control in health as authoritative, definitive, and exclusive; the syndrome of professional dominance which devalues lay activity in established domains of professional expertise.[5]

The almost exclusive concept of professional health intervention has, at the very least, deflected interest in lay interventions by encouraging the view that such practices are dangerous, scientifically unsubstantiated, and associated with superstitious and parochial mentalities. In effect, this view holds that self-care in health is a folk practice, culture-bound and "indigenous," riddled with absurd and ineffectual remedies, rampantly empirical, contributing on occasion to unnecessary delays in seeking professional care and often implicated in the failure of laypersons to follow prescribed medical regimens.[6] Self-care, so viewed, is considered a vestigial or at best a residual health function in the wake of the growth of "modern medicine" and is to be avoided and deplored.

A second factor which may have obfuscated the realities of self-care behavior was noted by Lois Pratt.[7] She suggests that the popular sociological theory, which holds that increased industrialization, technology, and the growing complexity of the social system have eliminated many previous social functions of the family, including health care, may be misleading. The interpretive error here is the inference that increased specialized health services, outside the lay domain, amount to substitution rather than supplementation or additional service. As applied to health, this functional theory fails to account for shifts in morbidity patterns which, in turn, may not be reflected in demands for professional intervention. Care of some forms of chronic disease—hypertension, mental illness, diabetes, for example—surely requires a high proportion of lay (individual and family) care relative to professional care. Pratt's review[8] of a rather modest research literature on self-care provides a reasonable basis for hypothesizing that self-care behavior has been and continues to be a substantial factor in health care. Several English studies, summarized by Fry, indicate that self-care practices are nearly universal among patients, and Fry concludes that "without self-care any system of health care would be swamped."[9] But it is clear that our knowledge of the extent and variation of self-care practice is fragmentary, and will require much national and cross-cultural inquiry using uniform definitions and observational standards heretofore lacking. Later chapters of this volume discuss such research needs from several perspectives.

Although the extent and effectiveness of present self-care practices is insufficiently known, it is clear that laypersons do retain civil rights as to self-diagnosis and self-treatment. While medical practice acts usually establish the grounds of exclusiveness in the practice of medicine and surgery, these regulations concern only the performance of healing acts for compensation, gain, or reward, received or expected. Thus, by default, the self-healing or self-care medical activity remains a virtually unchallenged civil right of all citizens.[10] This is not to say that laypersons enjoy equality with licensed practitioners regarding access to supporting medical technology such as narcotic and other restricted drugs, hospital privileges, and malpractice insurance. But aside from these specific interdictions, there appear to be no legal constraints on what a layperson can undertake to self-provide in medical care. The most crucial limitations in self-care functioning stem from the motivation, knowledge, custom, and competence of the individual.

Definitions and Illustrations

At the root of many debates on the role of self-care—and the Copenhagen conference was no exception—is the lack of a universally agreed definition of the term. Although semantic confusion (e.g., between self-care, self-help, medical care, health care) undoubtedly operates, differences in the definer's discipline, special interests, professional goals, and political orientation appear to contribute as well. To achieve a common definition may be possible only at the cost of losing the precision required for significant analytic research. On the other hand, at the present level of exploration and debate, diverse "working definitions" can stimulate thought about various perspectives on self-care. This strategy was adopted at the Copenhagen conference, by means of an opening statement, which offered a broad perspective on the layperson's role in primary health care, and through background papers.

Among the formulations presented in the latter, Harvey Smith defined self-care as "an action taken by the consumer or patient, to reduce, to the degree possible, incremental debilitation resulting from chronic disease."[11] A similar definition was given by Lowell

Levin: ". . . a process whereby a layperson functions on his/her own behalf in health promotion and prevention and in disease detection and treatment at the level of the primary health resource in the health care system."[12] John Fry identified four roles for self-care: health maintenance; disease prevention; self-diagnosis, self-medication, and self-treatment; and patient participation in professional care (use of services).[13] In addition to the specific behaviors these formulations describe, they all have some underlying common premises: that self-care is a voluntary, self-limited, non-organized, universal, varying complex of behaviors evolved through a mixture of socializing and cognitive experiences. Self-care is an indigenous phenomenon, wholly outside the framework of professional health resources, although obviously influenced by the nature of the social institutions of care, and the context of economic, social, and political structures. Thus, self-care may be viewed as involving both the continuous substrate of behavior (custom, life style) and discrete or episodic actions (self-diagnosis, self-treatment). The evaluative process is largely pragmatic in nature, based on criteria personally perceived as relevant; criteria which may or may not conform to professional criteria of effectiveness.

Self-care can also be viewed as a decision-making process which involves self-observation, symptom perception and labeling, judgment of severity, and choice and assessment of treatment options. Analytic models for the study of illness behavior, such as that proposed by Fabrega,[14] offer theoretical frameworks for conceptualization of the process as a problem-solving system.

An additional function of self-care was proposed at the Copenhagen conference: contributing to the social accountability of the health professions. This may occur at several levels; the first at that of the personal use of professional resources. Clearly, the individual's perspective on his own competence to self-diagnose and self-treat contributes toward his decision to seek professional assistance for a given problem.[15] Of course, this may be simply a matter of market conditions. A second level of accountability and control occurs in the context of the patient-professional interaction. Expectations of patients and their entry and performance in the "patient role" reflect complex judgments regarding the efficacy, appropriateness, and satisfactions of the service.[16] Social inhibitions on the effective and full exercise of these judgments are an important part of the need and justification for self-care education, as discussed in a later section of this book.

Finally, there is the level of public interest, decision-making, and political action in health affairs. These reflect individual and group perspectives on the functions, organization, management, extent, availability, quality control, and costs of professional health care undertakings. Consumerism has recently emerged as a substantial factor in health policy and practice, pointing to both the actual and potential lay impact on the functioning of professional health resources.[17] This level of lay or public influence and action in health, of course, broadly reflects a variety of self-care competencies as perceived by many sections of the population.

The operational objectives of self-care can serve as another dimension of definition: i.e., self-care directed at: one's own health; the health of one's family or group; and the health of one's community. This level of approach to self-care introduces the dimension of social functions (fiduciary relationships in the care of the family or group) and political relationships (in the case of community action, e.g., participation in decisions regarding allocation of health resources). It is clear that self-care should not be viewed in terms of self-interest alone, since (1) health problems are multifactorial in origin and effects; their solution usually requires some degree of social manipulation or change; and (2) individuals perform multiple social roles, which offer opportunities for and often demand the application of self-care skills to the needs of others. Personal behavior in self-care is a health resource whose effects aggregate in family, extended social groups, and community life. In this sense, self-care behavior can be defined as a characteristic attribute of whole populations; as a level or element in social competence to cope with health and disease, complementary or alternative to the professional health resources.

In summary, there was agreement in Copenhagen that the divergent perspectives on self-care, which reflect semantic, cultural, and motivational differences, require a taxonomy of sufficient breadth to allow comprehensive ordering of observations. Such a classification scheme could make possible cross-national and cross-cultural comparisons and avoid arbitrary or preemptory labeling. The simple questions: "What is self-care?" and "How do we know self-care when we see it?" cannot be fully answered by direct observations stemming from solely professional criteria of health behavior. Like Molière's character who did not realize he had been talking prose for forty years—much self-care is not labeled as such but is found in a wide range of naturally occurring phenomena.

The Mixture of Self-Care and Professional Care

Society as an ecosystem is a reality we can better sense than measure. Tools of observation and strategies of analysis provide only partial clues to the relationship of components to system. In looking at health and health care the task of differentiating interactive components is complicated by some difficulties of an ethological nature. One is the relationship of health care to broad cultural characteristics in a given society. To isolate the specific components of a health care system apart from the cultural context is hazardous. Cross-cultural comparisons are also difficult for similar reasons. Efforts to isolate and relate self-care behavior to professional care are further hampered by a prevailing lack of agreement on definitions and differences about whether it is a significant component of health care as a whole. As a result, the Copenhagen meeting had to fall back on impressions derived from personal clinical experience, buttressed by a meager body of research, diverse in focus and disparate in study base and methods.[18]

One can, however, discern a general consensus on trends in self-care from the studies cited by Pratt,[19] Fry,[20] and Kirscht,[21] which suggest that perhaps 75 percent or more of health care is undertaken without professional intervention. The difficulty comes in placing self-care behavior within the context of the care options available to an individual or group over time, which covers a wide range of health behavior. Several studies[22,23] are exemplary in one aspect or another, but fall short of providing the requisite comprehensive design.

At this point we are limited to the observation that in relation to professional intervention in health, self-care includes behaviors which both supplement and substitute for professional health care procedures. Indeed, it may be historically more accurate and more practical to state the proposition in reverse: that professional health care procedures include those which supplant or substitute for self-care behavior. Lois Pratt summarized several major studies which tend to support this view:

> A large amount of illness and disability are cared for exclusively by the family without professional assistance. An English study of general

> practice estimated that there is a hard core of three percent of persons who consistently do not obtain professional care for seven years or more (Kessel and Shepard, 1965). [A study by White et al., 1961] estimated that 75 out of every 100 adults in United States, England and Wales will experience some illness or injury during a month . . . [and that] about two-thirds of those experiencing an illness take care of it without professional consultation. The family's dominant role in caring for illness is brought out even more sharply in . . . [A study by Alpert et al., 1967] of a month of illnesses among low income families [in the U.S.]: medical help was sought in only 12 percent of the 834 symptoms identified by the families. The ratio of medically non-attended symptoms was seven to one. . . .
>
> Even among U.S. civilians who sustain injuries during the course of a year which are serious enough to require activity restriction for a day or more, 14 percent . . . receive no professional medical attention (HEW, 1970).[24]

It is clear, then, from a diverse research literature, that self-care practices are particularly prominent at the level of primary care both in terms of health practices and health judgments. In the view of primary medical practitioners, however, there remains a significant level of demand for services which might be but are not now being effectively self-treated. In the Dunnel and Cartwright study, the authors reported that "Half the doctors [surveyed] thought that at least a quarter of their consultations were for conditions which people could treat themselves."[25] A study by Williamson,[26] also in Britain, showed similar results. Using a 1974 Department of Health morbidity survey of general practice, Williamson sent these data to a series of general practitioners for judgment as to those diseases for which medical care had something to offer; those diseases that could be supplemented by self-care; and those conditions in which self-care could be substituted. Excluding trauma, pregnancy, cancer, and the like, Williamson found that approximately 25 percent of the illness episodes seen in general practice were believed by the practitioner to be ones in which self-care could be *substituted* entirely; and that 15 to 18 percent of the listed illnesses could achieve a better result if *supplemented* by self-care.

It is clear that the optimal balance between self-care and professional care is not easily determined. Some pertinent findings do emerge, however: (1) The decision to contact the professional care-giver is largely but not totally, at the initiative of the patient;[27]

(2) it is often, further, the product of a lay referral process;[28] (3) a good part of the care for a given complaint takes place prior to sharing responsibility with the physician; (4) treatment decisions may be patient-determined (particularly patient requests for prescriptions); (5) patients vary with regard to compliance with the professional treatment plan; and (6) patients habitually participate in evaluation of professional care (efficacy and outcomes).

What exists, then, at the micro-level, the doctor-patient dyad, is a highly complex, interacting amalgam of functions, some complementary, some substitutive. Recognition and conceptualization of the doctor-patient relationship in these terms as a two-way process, led one observer to propose a contractual procedure which would clarify and stipulate the responsibilities of both parties. Of course, the relationship is still unequal in power, adversarial as well as cooperative, and often conflicting with regard to expectations. Both empirical studies and much sociological theory describe influential and predisposing factors—e.g., patient's perception of illness, sick role, the influence of culture; the physician's "apostolic function"; the personality and attitudes of the patient; the specifics of the "transaction" including the legitimizing function of the doctor; and the compliance function of the patient.[29,30,31,32,33] The fiduciary character of the doctor-patient relationship is emphasized as one keystone. To strengthen the patient's trust is a major goal, achievable, as one writer puts it, through "conversation . . . education . . . or training: of the patient by the doctor to his 'standards and beliefs'."[34] Few would argue for blind faith; indeed, many practitioners agree that an appropriate degree of patient independence at appropriate phases in the therapeutic relationship is beneficial. How much, when, and where and how patients should be encouraged or helped to achieve more control over their situation is not, however, agreed. The characteristics of the patient, the nature and stage of illness, the doctor's style, are all considered factors in the professional's decision regarding an appropriate model. On the whole, the literature and theoretical perspectives on the doctor-patient relationship tend to ignore the possibilities of patient manipulation of the relationship as a major protective device in maintaining personal integrity, in establishing patient priorities and values, and in controlling undesired iatrogenic effects. The concept of patient rights in the doctor-patient relationship, and techniques to achieve a more effective decision-making input, are now the subject of a plethora of popular books.[35,36]

At the macro-level of community health, the desirable balance or mixture of lay/professional intervention has in recent decades been widely discussed in economic, political, organizational, and ideological terms. Consumer challenges to professional control in health escalated during the 1960s and, while waning in intensity since then, remain as an important demand for a role in health decision-making, even institutionalized in America[37] and Britain.[38] Present arrangements for orderly involvement of laypersons in public health decisions reflect, on the whole, a productive experience of lay participation in health services. However, the differentiation of lay and professional functions has sometimes become blurred in practice. Thus, the Danaceau report of four in-depth case studies on consumer involvement in the planning and operation of health services concludes: "Clear cut distinctions between policy (a board matter) and administration (a staff matter) exist only in bureaucratic theory, not in reality."[39]

As is true with other dimensions of self-care, one can expect wide cultural variation in lay initiatives in health policy and health systems operations. But for several and diverse reasons discussed in the chapter to follow, it appears that one can discern a general support of the view expressed by Freidson in his discussion on limiting professional autonomy: ". . . it is essential that in order to protect the public interest the lay public dominate the formation of policy decisions, guiding the planning of services and the determination of the economic and social terms of the performance of work."[40]

References

[1] Horace Miner, "Body Ritual Among the Nacirema," *American Anthropologist* 59 (June 1956), pp. 503–507.

[2] L. Riddick Lynch (ed.), *The Cross-Cultural Approach to Health Behavior* (Rutherford, New Jersey: Fairleigh Dickinson University Press, 1969).

[3] John Williamson, *Healthward Care (The Semantics of Self-Care)*, Department of General Practice, Guy's Hospital Medical School, 15 St. Thomas Street, London, S.E.1, England. Unpublished manuscript, p. 6.

[4] Marjorie A.C. Young, "Review of Research Studies Related to Health Education Practice (1961–1966): What People Know, Believe and Do About Health," *Health Education Monographs*, Number 23, 1967.

[5] Eliot Freidson, *Professional Dominance: The Social Structure of Medical Care* (New York: Atherton Press, 1970).

[6]National Analysts, Inc., *A Study of Health Practices and Opinions* (Springfield, Virginia: National Technical Information Service, U.S. Department of Commerce, June, 1972).

[7]Lois Pratt, "The Significance of the Family in Medication," *Journal of Comparative Family Studies* IV, No. 1 (Spring 1973), pp. 13–31.

[8]*Ibid.*

[9]John Fry, "Self Care: Its Place in the Total Health Care System." A report by an independent working party, September 1973, 15 pp. (Mimeographed.)

[10]In the United States the practice of health services is covered by the general state statutes. An example is Title 20–9 of the Connecticut General Statutes. Formally, there is no such legal entity as "self-care" or "self-help," only the "practice of medicine or surgery." Regulations concerning the latter have to do with performance of acts for compensation, gain, or reward, received or expected.

[11]C. Harvey Smith, "Some Thoughts About Self-Care Education," paper submitted to the Symposium on the Role of The Individual in Primary Health Care, Institute of Social Medicine, University of Copenhagen, Copenhagen, Denmark, August 11–15, 1975. (Mimeographed.)

[12]Lowell S. Levin, "The Layperson as the Primary Care Practitioner," *Public Health Reports* 91 (May-June 1976), pp. 206–210.

[13]John Fry, "Role of the Patient in Primary Health Care: The Viewpoint of the Medical Practitioner," background paper for the Symposium on the Role of The Individual in Primary Health Care, Institute of Social Medicine, University of Copenhagen, Copenhagen, Denmark, August 11–15, 1975. (Mimeographed.)

[14]Horacio Fabrega, Jr., "Toward a Model of Illness Behavior," *Medical Care* XI, No. 6 (November-December 1973), pp. 470–484.

[15]Karen Dunnel and Ann Cartwright, *Medicine Takers, Prescribers and Hoarders* (London and Boston: Routledge and Kegan Paul, 1972).

[16]Marshall H. Becker (ed.), "The Health Belief Model and Personal Health Behavior," *Health Education Monographs* 2, No. 4, (Winter 1974).

[17]Eli Glogow, "Community Participation and Sharing in Control of Public Health Services," *Health Services Reports* 88 (May 1973), pp. 442–448.

[18]See "Self-Care in Health" Annotated Bibliography.

[19]Pratt, *op. cit.*

[20]Fry, "Self Care," *op. cit.*

[21]John P. Kirscht, "The Health Belief Model and Illness Behavior," *Health Education Monographs* 2, No. 4 (Winter 1974), pp. 387–408.

[22]Poul A. Pedersen, "Varighed fra sygdoms begyndelse til henvendelse til praktiserende læge," *Ugeskr. Læg.* 138, No. 32 (2 August 1976), pp. 1962–1966.

[23]Dunnel and Cartwright, *op. cit.*

[24]Pratt, *op. cit.*, pp. 15–16.

[25]Dunnel and Cartwright, *op. cit.*, p. 121.

[26]John Williamson reported this study at the Symposium.

[27] K. Roghmann and Robert Haggerty, "The Diary as a Research Instrument in the Study of Health and Illness Behavior," *Medical Care* X (March-April 1972), pp. 143–163.

[28] Stanislav Kasl, "Social Psychological Characteristics Associated with Behaviors which Reduce Cardiovascular Risk," in *Applying Behavioral Science to Cardiovascular Risk,* Allan Enelow and Judith Henderson (eds.), proceedings of a conference, Seattle, Washington, June 17–19, 1974. (New York: American Heart Association, 1975).

[29] D.D. Etzwiler, "The Contract for Health Care," *Journal of the American Medical Association* 224 (May 14, 1973), p. 1034.

[30] Samuel W. Bloom, *The Doctor and His Patient* (New York: Russell Sage Foundation, 1963).

[31] Michael Balient, *The Doctor, His Patient and His Illness* (New York: International Universities Press, Inc., 1957).

[32] Ann Cartwright, *Patients and Their Doctors* (New York: Atherton Press, 1967).

[33] T.S. Szasz and M.H. Hollander, "A Contribution to the Philosophy of Medicine: The Basic Models of the Doctor-Patient Relationship," *Archives of Internal Medicine* 97 (May 1956), pp. 585–592.

[34] Balient, *op. cit.,* p. 239.

[35] Arthur Levin, *Talk Back to Your Doctor* (New York: Doubleday and Company, Inc., 1975). See also, "Self-Care in Health" Annotated Bibliography.

[36] Keith W. Sehnert, *How to Be Your Own Doctor (Sometimes)* (New York: Grosset and Dunlap, 1975). For a cogent analysis of the apparent contretemps in being an informed patient, see: M.J. Bloar and G.W. Horobin, "Conflict and Conflict Resolution in Doctor Patient Interactions," in *A Sociology of Medical Practice,* Caroline Cox and Adrianne Mead (eds.), (London: Collier-MacMillan, 1975), pp. 271–284.

[37] 93rd United States Congress, *Public Law 93–641, An Act.*(Washington, D.C.: U.S. Government Printing Office, 1975).

[38] Secretary of the State for Social Services, *National Health Service Reorganization: England* (London: Her Majesty's Stationery Office, 1972).

[39] Paul Danaceau, *Consumer Participation in Health Care: How It's Working* (Arlington, Virginia: Human Services Institute for Children and Families, Inc., May 1975), p. 4.

[40] Eliot Freidson, *Profession of Medicine* (New York: Dodd, Mead and Co., Inc., 1973), p. 374.

CHAPTER III

New Impetus for Self-Care

Public Interest in Self-Care

While acknowledging the existence of self-care as a universal if highly variable attribute of all societies, participants in the Copenhagen Symposium were not agreed on the proposition that self-care is becoming the subject of new or significantly greater public interest. One participant stated: "I think that the use of the word popular . . . may have different connotations to different people. I think self-care has been popular. I don't think it is now a popular movement or popular phenomenon, but it has always been popular and varied in different societies." Other participants found evidence for increased interest in self-care, but were not sure that this signified more than a fashionable trend. Skepticism was expressed about the promotion of self-care with missionary zeal and the danger that public expectations might be raised that are incapable of being fulfilled. An American participant ". . . didn't want to be any part of [supporting] the sort of general feeling that doctors are going to give all the power to the people and the people are all going to be better for it . . . [have a] better self-concept and be more dignified."

Others expressed cautious optimism that development in health self-care is in fact a reality; and that therefore the challenge to professionals is to decide if, what, and how to provide technical, research, and educational support to improve or expand it.

Early in the Symposium proceedings it became clear that the mixture of cultures, disciplines, and beliefs in the group resulted in differing views of the current importance of the phenomenon. Consensus was not attained on the notion that self-care currently has a strong impact on individual and community health. Although most participants acknowledged that new demands for self-care in some areas of health have emerged, questions remained about how to interpret these demands.

Are we, for example, witnessing mere isolated episodes of concern that reflect specific, limited failures in the professional health care system? Will that interest decline or fade altogether when those specific failures are corrected? Or, on the contrary, do these apparently isolated episodes of self-care activity reflect more fundamental changes in social assumptions and expectations? Can the acceleration of self-care undertakings on a broad and pervasive basis be realistically anticipated? Is the urgency to consider self-care at this time real or is it simply an artifact of political motivation and/or professional frustration? Regardless of whether or not the status of self-care as a factor in health has changed, why has its professional recognition been so long delayed? Why have professionals had so little interest in what is going on outside the professional health care domain?

In the absence of research, discussion of these basic questions could yield only speculative answers. But, as the Symposium demonstrated, such speculation can encourage insight and sensitivity to the issues, and can lead to a research strategy on self-care which takes into account political, economic, and social-psychological dimensions as well as the more traditional outcomes of health care.

As the first international symposium on self-care, the Copenhagen meeting provided a productive environment for the disclosure and refinement of attitudes and beliefs through the dialectic of sharp challenges and responses.

In discussing the primary question of why self-care draws greater attention at the present time, the participants advanced several factors thought responsible for this rising interest. Not necessarily in order of priority, these were: (1) the "de-mystification" of primary medical care; (2) "consumerism" and popular demands for increased self-control—related to anti-technology, anti-authority sentiments; (3) changes in life-style and rising educational levels; (4) lay concern with regard to perceived abuses in medical care; and (5) the lack of availability of professional services.

Let us discuss these factors in sequence.

1. The professional monolith of medicine, with its inherent attributes of guildism, monopoly of diagnostic and treatment functions, and social control, has been carefully delineated.[1] Indeed, sociologists describe medicine as an almost impenetrable fortress, with little expectation that it will be effectively breached.[2] This analysis may be valid in reference to the "medicalization" of politics,[3] on the one hand, and the structural control of secondary (consultative) medical care, on the other.

However, primary health care appears to be one of the domains most accessible to lay activity; or, otherwise stated, one least successfully dominated by professional expertise. All the complex dimensions of this phenomenon have not yet been fully studied or understood. Some seminar participants noted that the profile of lay involvement at the primary care level is uneven and variable; some segments of the population demand training in additional technical-medical skills and responsibility, others less so. In general, however, the participants agreed that the modal level of lay activity and demands for increased self-care may be moving upward. Also noted was a general, if diffuse, rise in society's mistrust of professional motives as these affect the public interest; and broad public concern about the depersonalizing effects of technology.

Concurrently, expressions of public unease about the diminishing areas of personal control, as for example in the civil rights movement in the U.S., have resulted in dramatic confrontations with previously unchallenged professional policies and practices. These social trends have led to unprecedented public disclosure of inadequacies and inequities in professional services, including medical services at the primary and neighborhood levels. One solution to these problems has been the concept of new health careers, and the substantial expansion of efforts to redistribute primary care by assigning functions to others than the medically trained.[4]

Green and Welin describe this phenomenon: "Once some [medical] functions had been wrested from the medical profession, the veil lifted from a variety of medical procedures. . . . It became much easier then to transfer more of these functions . . . to the consumer or patient himself."[5] Arcane or monopolistic professional expertise has been challenged and the limits of medicine scrutinized.

2. Changes in life-styles appear to be another source of current interest in self-care. Massive cultural changes since World War II, and especially in the last decade, include shifting values, greater non-conformity and less commitment to traditional roles in the population, concern with more personal independence in decision-making, a recasting of traditional sex roles, and expectations for achievement and personal fulfillment less competitive and materialistic than in the past.

More specifically, the de facto lowering of the age of majority seems typical of a changing status for children and youth in North America and Western Europe. Overall, such life-style changes seem to provide a psycho-social milieu hospitable to and compatible with self-care ideas. Increased assumption of self-care responsibility might contribute to building self-assurance and an improved self-concept; to reducing dependence on social institutions; to increasing family cohesiveness; and to renewed emphasis on health behaviors in a broad context of social priorities.

Rising educational levels and increasing access to technical information through multiple media sources also were seen as key factors in stimulating effective demand for self-care. Although there is little evidence that people generally apply more discriminant criteria in processing health information, it seems obvious that opportunities to exercise personal judgment have increased. Simultaneously, increased population mobility has reduced the historical importance of primary reference groups as contributing factors in individual decision-making. Thus, sociologically speaking, the individual may have become more isolated; more dependent on his own decision-making capability and experience, and less on legitimating social processes.[6] Several participants saw rising educational levels as a major factor in increased public demand for self-care knowledge and skills. There are, however, no data on which to base a conclusion that effective demand for self-care is a function of educational attainment. However, one can note in this connection the rising market demand for the burgeoning list of books and treatises designed to enhance self-care knowledge and skills. Such materials have always had a modest but steady market (Tennent's *Every Man His Own Doctor* had five editions between 1734 and 1737),[7] but the current self-care materials are extensive in subject coverage, appear to be increasingly sophisticated,[8] and enjoy wide circulation.

It is probable that the public consciousness with regard to self-care has achieved somewhat higher levels in recent years in the U.S. than in other countries represented at the Copenhagen Symposium. The women's movement has focused national attention on the quality of care received by women in a male-dominated medical care system. Specifically it has been charged that women are subjected to a wide range of abuses, physical, psychological, and civil.[9] Gynecological and obstetrical services are of particular concern. Recommendations for change center on the woman herself, in terms of increased knowledge of her anatomy, physiology, risk status for sex-related morbidities, and techniques of self-examination. The latter emphasis has moved self-care across the line from supplementation to substitutive behavior. Heretofore, self-observation had been limited to breast self-examination, a procedure professionally encouraged as valuable routine lay procedure. Self-examination of the vagina by speculum, however, a recent and unprecedented incursion into the professional domain, has caused widespread debate.[10] The speculum, in effect, became a symbol of a more general intent of women to achieve more humane, unbiased, and efficacious medical care even if this requires challenging lay-professional jurisdictional taboos. Women's clinics in America now provide training in self-care practices (including birth control techniques and abortion counseling) and offer, through the mutual-aid process, training in assertiveness vis-à-vis the use of professional resources.[11]

The point was made in Copenhagen that a major impetus to self-care may arise from situations in which professional health resources are completely lacking. Thus, the group was reminded that ". . . 80 percent of populations in third world countries have no access to professional health care whatsoever. So there you can say that self-care is most popular." However, the total absence of professional health resources (as defined by western science) does not mean a vacuum of other specialized resources (e.g., shamans, witch doctors, priests) who provide medical care at levels of effective demand as high or higher than in developed societies. Demands for increased competence in self-care may be great in situations where the population perceives the "professional" resources as inadequate, ineffective, or dangerous. Such demands are clearly influenced by many factors not yet charted or fully understood. For example, demands for self-care skills could increase dramatically when a population totally dependent on professional care suddenly finds itself deprived of that resource and unlikely to replace it.[12] Thus, severe, sustained, or total reduction of health personnel during wartime might stimulate interest in self-care. But as of this writing, the functional relationship of the availability of professional services to demends for self-care is still unclear.

Professional Interest in Self-Care

Participants in the Copenhagen Symposium certainly were not of a common mind with regard to all the potential benefits or liabilities of self-care. But there was evident a common interest in questions of self-care as it has or might have impact on (1) the status of personal health in an era of chronic illness; (2) the conservation of professional health resources and the containment of costs; and (3) the achievement of a health care system limited by and accountable to the public.

Self-Care and Chronic Disease

The prevalence of illness in the population suggests that an individual's chance of being totally symptom-free on any given day are remote. In summarizing research on this point, Zola concludes that some form of illness is the statistical norm.[13] However, there are no satisfactory data on how illnesses are distributed in terms of severity (including social as well as medical consequences) as they correlate with levels of professional health care intervention. There is likewise little knowledge of the nature and degree of chronic illness which has never been professionally managed. It would be clearly helpful to have data on this point as a basis for understanding lay activity in chronic disease care. However, some data, reviewed by Pratt, indicate that lay involvement in long-term care, both with and without professional input, represents a significant factor, especially in convalescent care and care of the bedfast elderly.[14]

Existing data on lay self-care in chronic disease suggest that it may have magnitude, but do not throw light on the character of lay performance throughout various phases of the natural history of chronic disease. Knowledge of lay behavior with regard to chronic disease is generally limited to the later stages of treatment, where professional assessment of patient needs has clarified the patient's role and the role of the family, e.g., the importance of lay management skills, such as insulin taking, blood pressure monitoring, and diet. Lay functions in chronic disease control at the prodromal or prepathology and the presymptomatic stages must also be considered as a potential factor in applying preventive and ameliorative knowledge and techniques. The central interest in the Copenhagen discussions of self-care in chronic disease focused on its role in the reduction and control of disability and dependence. It was observed that chronic disease constitutes a clear and comprehensive model for self-care practice, an opportunity for laypersons to develop extensive self-care skills on a continuous and progressive basis. As a design for purposeful self-care education, the chronic disease model was noted as an effective meeting-place for the interaction of social and clinical self-care skills. The effective control of chronic disease is helping to define the limitations of medicine, and the crucial contribution individuals and families can make.

Conservation of Professional Health Resources and Cost Containment

At Copenhagen, the economic implications of self-care appeared to be of special interest to planners and health practitioners in countries where there is no national health service, where fee-for-service and the absence of a resources allocation plan cause grave inequities and abuses in health care delivery. One participant summed up this view by asking: "Do we need self-care in the welfare state, or is it needed only in countries with a capitalist system?" Another participant raised the contrary speculation that citizens of a welfare state may abuse the privilege of free access to medical care and would benefit by a self-care capability. The conservation of professional health resources through self-care was a motif of major interest to the U.S. participants. There was also wide interest in this aspect of self-care among participants both from countries with national health systems, and from those with mixed private/public systems.

Interest in the economic implications of self-care was stimulated by observations of epidemiologists[15] and health economists.[16] Their analysis of data on the contribution of medical care to life expectancy and to the reduction of major morbidity trends, emphasized that medical care has relatively modest effects.[17] This is not to gainsay medicine's therapeutic benefits, but rather to emphasize its historically limited impact on the course of many serious infectious diseases such as tuberculosis, scarlet fever, and cholera. Although this finding is by no means a recent discovery, its enunciation at a time of severe economic pressure draws attention to the cost/benefit analysis of human services.

Some observers have suggested shifting the major investment in manipulations of the professional resource toward an approach which includes a significant effort toward improving the health competence of laypersons. The labor-intensive character of health services, particularly in meeting the increased demands for preventive care and chronic disease management, suggests a new look at the lay resources as the *primary,* primary health care resource. This is not to argue that achieving a more individually responsible and self-active society would immediately result in cost containment or reduction. The mounting of a purposeful educational effort to raise and maintain self-care competency levels would undoubtedly be expensive. Other aspects of cost involvement must also be taken into account; costs of the laypersons' time, treatment costs, and iatrogenic effects. But there are crucial differences between investments in lay and professional health resources. The lay investment may be potentially more progressive in the sense that there are inherent economies in the concept of consumer as self-provider. Skills possessed by consumers are immediately available as productive output, self-adjusting and discriminately applied according to self-observed effectiveness. Self-care skills can accrue, become assimilated as coping skills, and passed on to others through the processes of socialization. Thus, over time, self-care skills can have a multiplier effect.

Several participants suggested other, perhaps more immediate bases for interest in the economic potentials of self-care. These relate to the inefficient use of professional resources, especially the primary care physician. Reflecting on their own experience, general physicians at the Symposium corroborated findings reported by investigators (Williamson, Dunnel and Cartwright, *op. cit.*) that much of their work involved services which the patient could have provided for himself. Some of their patients over-used services, as measured by professional criteria of appropriateness. Failures in patient compliance also were cited as a factor that influences efficiency and, consequently, raised the cost of care to both patient and provider. While acknowledging the complexity of these behaviors, these general practitioners believed that improvement of self-care competency in their patients would be a useful innovation. Sehnert's experience as cited at the Symposium indicated that an adult self-help educational program reduced the number of telephone calls to the doctor, lowered patient anxieties, improved patients' ability to describe their problems, and reduced patient "estrangement" from the medical profession.

Hard data are not yet available on whether self-care is also a cost-saving strategy, either through its supplementary or substitutive role; or through increasing the efficiency of professional practice. It was emphasized that shifts in lay competency levels, however slight, represent a weighted change many times exceeding comparable changes in the professional domain. Cost accounting of the effects of self-care, therefore, should be designed for measurement on a regional or national scale. Accounting procedures would have to acknowledge variations in self-care competence levels among different ethnic, social, and age groups. Such studies could incorporate observations of systems and organizational changes (e.g., manpower reallocation, functional revisions) as these are affected by shifts in self-care competence. Specific research designs were proposed in accordance with these goals (see Chapter V).

Achievement of a Limited and Accountable Health Care System

An accountable health system, by definition, is one which is built on clear delineation of responsibility for policy decisions (public) and technical applications (professional). It is a technical support system which society defines and regulates in the public interest. As discussed earlier, a health care system of this character is an ideal yet to be achieved. Medicine is still profoundly self-controlling; there are few indications that it will capitulate before compelling arguments for democratization. Medical education remains essentially conservative and protective of professional values, roles, and social prerogatives despite various efforts to introduce consumer perspectives in medical education and practice. In contrast with previous strategies for change, Symposium participants emphasized that developing lay self-care competence has a powerful potential for deprofessionalizing the health care system. Using the conceptual frameworks of McKnight[18] and Illich,[19] this would include "demedicalizing" politics. Clearly the proponents of this view were asserting that democratization of health care is a major goal in its own right, quite apart from improving the health care system. In this sense, the proposed reform of the system would curtail and restrict its political influence and role to the provision of essential technical inputs.

Underlying this discussion was the belief that lay dependency on the health care system *qua* system, and lay dependency in personal care transactions, are similarly destructive of human integrity, dignity, and autonomy. It was argued that the loss of self-reliance and autonomy can seriously affect personal health, particularly in situations where patient initiative (e.g., self-observation for prevention and self-treatment for chronic disease) is crucial.

This argument for participant interest in self-care, like others previously cited, did not go unchallenged. Political, technical, and philosophical perspectives on self-care were so intermingled that no protagonist of self-care has a single *raison d'être* for supporting it. The varied motivations for interest in self-care are, of course, overlapping and interactive. Understanding requires sensitivity to all its contributing elements. As a first venture, limited by constraints of time and knowledge, the Copenhagen Symposium was an example of what may occur when self-care is discussed without an opportunity for full exposition and clarification of assumptions. A salubrious aspect of discussions of this kind, however, is their iterative character, which permits identification of basic themes as well as variations. There can be little doubt that the Symposium participants were impressed with the potential benefits of increased self-care competence. They were aware also that factors, wholly or in part outside the control of the medical care system, such as the prevalence of chronic disease and the rising costs of care, require solutions that must be implemented by the whole society, not just the health care segment.

The interest in self-care at Copenhagen was not merely the inevitability of its development, or its present technical state, or its possible development or evolution. Rather, interest in self-care reflected conviction that it embodies a complex of salient issues, organized around the portents of a major social change.[20] The trends toward increased self-care were viewed as a symptom of larger potential shifts in society's problems, priorities, and solutions—shifts which may not follow established precedents, or will simply perpetuate familiar institutions and patterns. In the instance of health care, a new partnership between layperson, practitioner, and scientist may be emerging with new and distinctive rules of procedure, control, and evaluation. The Symposium's attention was largely concentrated on the dimensions of these issues, and the research required to understand them.

References

[1] Irving K. Zola, "Medicine as an Institution of Social Control," in Caroline Cox and Adrianne Mead (eds.), *A Sociology of Medical Practice* (London: Collier-Macmillan, 1975), pp. 170–185.

[2] Eliot Freidson, *Profession of Medicine* (New York: Dodd, Mead and Co., Inc., 1973), pp. 381–382.

[3] John McKnight, "The Medicalization of Politics," paper presented to the Conference on Limits of Medicine, Davos, Switzerland (Gottlieb Duttweiler-Institute), March 1975. (Mimeographed).

[4] Harold B. Wise and Martin Cherkasky, *Neighborhood Medical Demonstration Project (Comprehensive Health Services Funding Request) Program Year B—January 1, 1969, to December 31, 1969* (New York: Montefiore Hospital and Medical Center, 1968), p. 330.

[5] Lawrence W. Green and Stanley H. Welin, "Research and Demonstration Issues in Self-Care: Measuring the Decline of Medicocentrism," paper presented to Conference on Self-Care Programs, National Center for Health Services Research and Development, Rockville, Maryland, March 25–26, 1976.

[6] Herbert Lionberger, *Adoption of New Ideas and Practices* (Ames, Iowa: The Iowa State University Press, 1964).

[7] John Tennent, *Every Man His Own Doctor or The Poor Planter's Physician* (Williamsburg, Va.: William Parks, 1734), republished by Printing and Patent Office, Williamsburg, Va., 1971.

[8] See "Self-Care in Health" Annotated Bibliography.

[9] Boston Women's Health Book Collective, Inc., *Our Bodies, Ourselves. A Book by and for Women* (New York: Simon and Schuster, 1971), p. 276.

[10] Ellen Frankfort, *Vaginal Politics* (New York: Bantam Books, 1972).

[11] Feminist Women's Health Centers, 746 South Crenshaw Boulevard, Los Angeles, California, 90005.

[12] The experience of several rural communities in Oregon, U.S.A., are examples of this situation. A program entitled, "Family and Self-Help Education Program," was especially useful in helping doctorless communities develop some health-care skills in the lay population. These programs were sponsored by the Oregon Regional Medical Program, Portland, Oregon.

[13] Irving K. Zola, "Culture and Symptoms: An Analysis of Patients' Presenting Complaints," in Caroline Cox and Adrianne Mead (eds.), *op. cit.*, p. 24.

[14] Lois Pratt, "The Significance of the Family in Medication," *Journal of Comparative Family Studies* IV, No. 1 (Spring 1973), p. 15.

[15] Thomas McKeown, *Medicine in Modern Society* (London: George Allen and Unwin, Ltd., 1965).

[16] Victor Fuchs, *Who Shall Live?* (New York: Basic Books, Inc., 1975).

[17] Negative effects of medical care also must be taken into account re: iatrogenic illness and nosocomial infection. An example: side effects of smallpox vaccination which may in some current circumstances (U.S. and U.K.) be contributing more problems than protection.

[18] McKnight, *op. cit.*

[19] Ivan Illich, *Medical Nemesis: The Expropriation of Health* (London: Calder and Boyars, Ltd., 1975).

[20] See Chapter IV.

CHAPTER IV

Self-Care in Health: An Emerging Social Movement?

In earlier chapters we have touched on some of the converging social forces and professional concerns that are currently renewing attention on self-care and self-help approaches and techniques as important components in health care and health maintenance. We have seen that these social and professional concerns arise from and are embedded in the broad social environment in which health care is provided. The drive toward an increase of self-care in health parallels similar movements of "consumerism" for enlarging the self-help component in other major fields of human endeavor—e.g., education—which are viewed as having become too highly technologized, or which depend too heavily upon the specialized attributes and training of a monopolistic professional elite. These broad movements toward consumerism seek, among other things, a lessening of dependence on the tutelage of all kinds of service professionals.

In such a broad context, health self-care is an especially powerful idea, because health needs are of such universal and personal concern. Poor health directly affects the individual, the family, and the society. The concepts that individual personal behavior can promote and maintain good health,[1] can help to overcome disease, that people have self-directing and self-healing powers that can be consciously mobilized and applied, are psychologically appealing as well as biologically appropriate. In the broadest sense, the biological drive for survival may be seen as providing the motivational basis for purposeful self-care by the individual.

The intimate relationship between somatic and psychic processes may make the natural impulse even stronger. If self-care can enhance physiological functioning, it will simultaneously heighten socio-psychological or subjective feelings of well-being. Since the latter correlate highly with self-confidence, with coping ability and social competence, increased self-care can reduce the individual's dependency on outside resources, including contacts with health professionals.

Viewed in this light, greater self-care in health could be a socially and personally attractive innovation of considerable power.

From the point of view of the individual, it would be consistent with psychological development, needs, and desires. From the social point of view, it would embody and express generally recognized ideals of democratic participation and the citizen's right to pursue life and happiness. Applied to the field of health, these social/political goals would encourage professionals and administrators to facilitate the widest possible participation of the individual in the maintenance of his own health and psychic well-being. It is generally recognized that a citizen has the right to pursue and attain personal satisfaction and happiness.

Achieving this ideal is bolstered by an accumulating body of research which indicates that personal responsibility for various health behaviors, and participation in various aspects of health care, is not merely an abstract and socially desirable "good," but is an active and characteristic requirement of effective health care.[2] Especially in view of the nature of much contemporary morbidity—the prevalent diseases of affluent societies, for example, the chronic disorders, substance abuse, obesity, mental disturbances—it seems appropriate and necessary for people to assume greater responsibility for their own health.

For those who suffer from a chronic disease—i.e., a long-term and disabling but not fatal or life-threatening condition (these constitute at least 75 percent of the current morbidity in advanced countries)—the conscious participation of the patient in his own care is generally thought essential to the realization of even narrowly viewed clinical goals. Deeper understanding and pursuit of an appropriate regimen of diet, medication, physical exercise, rest, and other everyday routines, require above all an effective level of interchange and cooperation between the physician and the patient. Such cooperation frequently requires understanding and help of persons in the immediate environment who are important to the patient, such as his spouse, children, or other members of the household.

The objectives of such enhanced cooperation/support are clearly to increase the coping ability and social competence of the patient. The enhancement of healing, recovery, and rehabilitation potentials by a psychically supportive social and interpersonal environment, or the setbacks that can occur in its absence, have been well-documented in studies of stress-related pathological states, and of long-term or chronic disease. Studies such as those of Thomas Holmes[3] and his associates, of the social-psychological history of TB patients, or the well-known studies of Hinkle and Plummer[4] of telephone workers, upwardly mobile executives, and other vulnerable populations, have given strong evidence for this important social-medical finding, which can now be stated as an accepted principle.

Thus, recovery from many morbid conditions and the maintenance of health depend on the "patient" assuming a great measure of responsibility for himself. His readiness and ability to do so may be greatly influenced by the nature of the available social/psychological supports.

Psychologically, self-care in health also may be viewed as a natural consequence of the wish of patients and their families to do something constructive when illness occurs, instead of remaining passive. As we have seen, self-care is important, sometimes indispensable in preventing, *treating,* or stabilizing some of the most prevalent and debilitating current illnesses. Even when self-care may not be appropriate, or when patients and their families wish to be completely passive and dependent, studies have shown that greater communication and mutual understanding between physician and patient facilitates patient recovery.

Thus, the bio-psychological individual impulses and the broad social forces that have been earlier mentioned now bring self-care in health to center stage as an important social phenomenon and a growing social movement. We will now discuss in greater detail the forces that are affecting the development of this movement and the broad issues that it poses.

Some Factors Promoting Self-Care

A number of participants in the Copenhagen Symposium expressed the view that increasing numbers of physicians, especially those in primary care, now believe that a good deal more responsibility can be turned over to patients and their families than has previously occurred or been thought desirable. In the area of drugs, diet, the monitoring of vital factors such as blood pressure, weight, dietary intake, rest, and recreation, a greater role for patients and their families is being tried in several countries, through physician or lay initiatives, or some combination of both.

A related set of concerns reported as promoting interest in self-care are those of administrators and planners of health services—

political scientists, economists, and government planners. Such factors as steeply mounting costs of health care, the heavy emphasis upon expensive technology, the increasing shortage and/or maldistribution of physicians in the face of rising popular demands, have necessitated a re-evaluation of the widespread modes of delivering health services in all types of settings—the individual offices of physicians, clinics, hospitals, and the exploration of alternative options.

In a recent paper, Dr. H. Mahler, Director-General of the World Health Organization, supported such a reassessment:

> What I am advocating, for the industrial as well as the developing world, is for the health Establishment to make a major effort to describe all the health problems and the alternative ways of dealing with them in an objective way and then to accept a national decision-making process based on this evidence.[5]

It has been known for some time that many of the complaints brought to the office of the primary health care physician are, from the standpoint of health professionals, trivial in nature. This does not mean that these complaints do not have an important psychological significance to those who present them. But for administrators and planners, who seek ways of economizing so that the time of physicians will be most appropriately employed for those patients whose complaints are most relevant to what professional skills can offer, the increasing use of self-care approaches is obviously attractive and worthy of serious study and consideration.

A third factor commented on by Symposium participants is the widespread initiative taken by various disadvantaged, stigmatized, needy persons in the population who form self-help or mutual aid groups for special health conditions and needs. These citizens perceive that their specific needs for health care, for education, financial support, or other social help are not being met by established institutions and professionals, and they come together either to provide for those needs directly, or to bring pressure so that they will be provided for by public authorities. The proliferation of self-help groups in the health field has helped to popularize the idea that lay persons can do something about their health and that of peers or those closely associated with them. That these groups are an enduring and growing phenomenon and that they perform important functions in health education and maintenance is well-documented in recent writings.[6] Parenthetically, the existence of such self-help groups poses an interesting and important question: whether they provide merely a substitute dependency for that of physicians and other health professionals. In other words, do patients who join self-help groups for such problems as alcoholism or obesity merely transfer their innate dependency from the health professional to the lay self-help groups? The question awaits further study and investigation.

These, then, are some additional social factors that are helping to bring about the present interest in self-care. In the authors' view, the many and growing currents of social-professional influence and concern have not yet coalesced so that health self-care has the status of a full-blown social movement. The early and probably irreversible signs are there, but it will require at least a decade or more of steady development and testing for self-care in health to become a truly influential and powerful force, beyond its current indigenous manifestations.

For it to do so, several interrelated developments may be important. Among them, we may cite the need for continuing systematic study and grappling with the implications of self-care. If such study and testing reveals that there are technical advantages in self-care approaches, then professionals will be called upon to expedite the disclosure and transfer of technological knowledge to the lay sector. Another requirement would be for the steady increase in spontaneous self-help groups in the health care sphere. As these movements grow, they can be expected to become increasingly assertive, sophisticated, and mutually supportive. They will communicate among one another, increasingly raise demands for access to education and technical information, and see themselves as vehicles for its dissemination.

Most important, the movement will require increased readiness and ability on the part of patients and their families to assume greater responsibility for their own care. This would necessitate both many social changes and a continuation of the trends already touched on, such as the increasing prevalence of chronic health problems, continuously rising costs of health care, and the increasing questioning of monopolistic professional expertise. The social changes will need to be in the areas of greater patient education and access to technical knowledge, and structural changes in health care systems to make this possible. As the present social trend continues, the "enlightened" patient can be expected to see self-care increasingly as a viable alternative.

The Symposium participants noted many signs which indicate that such changes are already existent, and that they will probably continue. As the self-care movement expands and matures, it will raise in sharp relief a number of important professional, philosophical, legal-ethical, administrative, and political issues. These have been briefly referred to, but will now be more specifically discussed.

Professional-Lay Relationship Issues

The movement for greater health self-care will in the first place be confronted by professional attitudes, and by the decisions of policy-makers, both of which will greatly influence its viability. For the movement to succeed, health professionals will have to find its goals and methodologies broadly compatible with the values under which they have traditionally functioned over the years. Nevertheless, *the issue must be squarely faced.* Self-care is based on a set of assumptions that differ *in some ways* from those of the professionally trained. It would be misleading to assume that self-care operates wholly *within* the framework of professional practices and beliefs, or that it merely offers a variant and possibly more effective way of carrying out the latter. Are the goals of professionals and those of lay persons with respect to the definition of health in fact identical or compatible? A possible source of conflict in this area arises from the reality that the criteria for what constitutes health and illness have been established almost exclusively by professionals. These criteria may or may not coincide with lay ideas and beliefs. "Healthy" for what? In what circumstances can the individual afford to define himself as ill, and become eligible for Parsons' famous moratorium of social responsibilities.

Physicians have the legal responsibility and function of defining and legitimating illness in many social situations, ranging from excusing absence from work, passing on eligibility for disability pensions, to certifying mental incompetency or inability to manage one's own affairs. While there is a certain rough agreement among similarly trained physicians on the criteria for those judgments, it is also clear that the judgments are relative and temporal, varying with social circumstances and needs.

With the development and expansion of self-care approaches, these criteria of health and illness, though traditionally evolved and applied by physicians in social decision-making, will be subject to searching re-examination. In this connection, we may cite examples from the experiences of lay health self-help groups, indicating that *their* criteria of illness and competence, and their prognostications about what ill or disabled patients can achieve, differ sharply from those of health professionals. Thus, there is a good deal of evidence that the parents of severely handicapped children (who are in a position to observe their handicapped child twenty-four hours a day), have been able to offer supplementary or alternative information and prognoses about what their children can attain or do, that have powerfully influenced or altered the judgments of professionals. It is clear that physicians' or health agencies' criteria of functioning or social competence, i.e., in severe physical disability, are not necessarily uniform, reliable, or accepted by the patients themselves.

Resistance by some health professionals to increased employment of self-care modes is to be expected for many reasons. In the first place, professionals may deplore or resist the perceived invasion of their areas of expertise and exclusivity. The extreme pole of such attitudes is that health professionals, particularly physicians, would be left with concern about their role and functions in relation to a developing self-care competence for the population. If self-care practices increasingly breach the professional domain of function, will there be anything left for the health professional, especially the primary care provider, to do? Stating it in this way consciously exaggerates the issue, but such concerns are already being voiced and may be one factor in the resistance that exists and that can be expected to deepen.

Some Symposium participants noted that primary care providers may indeed be called upon to transfer some of their present functions to patients and/or their families, but that they will then undertake alternative or supplementary functions, most likely education. But there will inevitably be a time lag before the professional primary care giver has had an opportunity to learn a new educational technology and to experience a new source of gratification in an educational relationship with patients rather than the traditional therapeutic one.

An additional concern expressed by physicians is that increased self-care will disrupt the doctor-patient relationship. It seems appropriate to point out in this connection that, if properly designed, self-care should serve to *enhance* rather than to hinder patient-physician contacts, since it would necessarily heighten the patients' feelings of independence and self-confidence. It is true that some models of physicians' expectations regarding their patients will have to change radically. Encouragement of and cooperation with "activated" or "energized" patients—i.e., patients who are at once more self-responsible and more demanding of knowledge—will become a goal of curative medicine, replacing the concept of the patient as a passive recipient of professional ministrations and skills. Some Symposium participants believed that such a shift will be beneficial to physicians as well as to patients, since the former will be more comfortable in the knowledge that self-care educated patients will be more self-protective and more able to share responsibility for the outcomes of medical care.

Another issue is that health professionals may perceive a direct threat from increased self-care to their *economic* position, especially in countries that lack a national health care system, such as the United States at present. Physicians, and other health professionals dependent on them, may perceive that self-care poses a threat to their unusually privileged economic status, as well as to their monopolistic possession of technical knowledge.

What must be kept in mind is that the development of self-care *itself* reflects fundamental changes in the health care requirements of society and its priorities, as well as the fact that many preventive, diagnostic, and therapeutic practices are increasingly amenable to self-care. The perceived threat, therefore, to traditional professional health care roles and functions, may be appropriately characterized as a diffuse discomfort associated with such changes. Generally, self-care may be or become a focal point for professional concern at the erosion of economic and social privilege.

An ironic countervalance to the above is the possibility that some professional primary care givers may perceive self-care as an opportunity to enhance their professional status, through transferring many routine tasks which carry only modest economic or social rewards. This perception might become more dominant as the trend to "specialize the generalist" gains momentum. Some may consider this a "dumping" process; others, a logical, indeed mandatory, step toward preserving the integrity of primary practice with results of benefits to both patient and practitioner.

Philosophical, Ethical, and Political Issues

More deeply, apart from such direct self-interest considerations, conscientious professionals may be expected to have reservations about self-care, which arise from their training, their values, and their philosophic outlook. It should be stressed that the major content and methodology of present-day medical education involves the role-model of the patient as a largely passive recipient of professional services. Technical procedures related to examination, history-taking, diagnosis, and finally treatment, emphasize the mystique of the omniscient technical expert and healer. Patients are usually not given access to their medical records; their questions are frequently met with discouraging cursoriness or superficiality. Many studies of medical student socialization point to the powerful influence such attitudes exert as they are embodied in the behavior of charismatic clinical instructors.

Further, principles like "do no harm" and the related concepts of the physician's responsibility summed up in the Hippocratic Oath may be expected to give rise to fears that self-care will cause more problems than it solves. Questions of how far in the direction of self-care a radical reorganization of the bases of primary health care should go, are not only natural, but reflect reasoned caution on the part of scientifically trained practitioners, who know the limits of their own skills; the transitory nature of health "facts"; and the requirement for constant reappraisal of the efficacy of both the theory and practice of preventive, diagnostic, and treatment procedures. Furthermore, there is yet to be established an acceptable and uniform standard of quality of professional technology and functions, let alone of lay self-care practices. One Symposium member cautioned that a critical assessment of current, professionally controlled primary care functions needs to be accomplished before their transfer to the lay domain.

Medical practitioners also are aware that the appropriateness of diagnosis and effectiveness of treatment are, to differing degrees, subject to the variance both of experience and of the situation. This aspect of the practitioner's caution with regard to self-care often is presented rather globally, and implies widespread skepticism of relevant lay coping experience in health, and of competence to judge and to act rationally.

It is clear that the concern for caution in promulgating self-care procedures cuts both ways; care in the selection of skills to be transferred in terms of their legitimate benefits; and care in the laypersons' preparations for their use.

It should be noted also that a pronounced shift toward self-care runs counter to broad tendencies in the society toward increased technological knowledge, expertise, and specialization. Professional skepticism about the interest as well as ability of lay people to perform purposeful and complex health actions on their own behalf is a natural and expected attitude that conforms with many accepted premises and values of our technological societies. Such concerns, skepticism or lack of trust, may, however, be reduced if self-care is viewed not simply as a natural, untutored activity, but as one that involves linkages and cooperation with physicians and other health professionals in a purposeful, mutually beneficial educational endeavor. Self-care is a concept with deep roots in the populist values of self-control and self-determinism. Its development will surely result in de-mystifying professional functions and may cause a rewriting of medicine's social charter. By definition a population competent in self-care would effect many more changes than the simple redistribution of the ratio of lay-professional technical functions. We can anticipate a profound impact as well on many previously unchallenged definitions and concepts of health and health behavior.

Given the rising popular demand for increased self-care, some Symposium participants expressed an additional concern that arises from a combination of professional and philosophic considerations. This is the possibility of co-optative behavior by professionals, who will seek to dominate and control the development of self-care initiatives by lay persons, thus compromising its viability, and the universality of its appeal. Professionals interested in the movement will need to tread a narrow line between proffering essential technical knowledge, education, and assistance on the one hand, and on the other avoiding the appearance or reality of monopolistic determination of either the content or the processes of self-care development.

Economic, Administrative, and Legal Issues

Growing consideration of self-care issues will stimulate identification and discussion of related questions of fundamental import to health professionals and planners. For example, at what levels, and by whom are basic policy decisions to be taken on matters that affect the health of individuals, groups, the whole society? The issues of who are the decision-makers, and upon what bodies of knowledge and experience are their decisions to be grounded, will be strongly involved in considerations of the greater incorporation of self-care in ongoing or altered health programs. Vigorous "consumer" oriented demands for participation in such important decision-making will unquestionably emerge. However, there was some concern expressed in Copenhagen that the development of self-care with a central emphasis on personal health behavior may tend to dilute or deflect interest in concerted social action when this is required to achieve individual and community health objectives. The concept and development strategies in self-care must be cast in terms sufficiently broad to include the political skills of consumerism while avoiding the politicization of self-care which could jeopardize its universality. Lay participation in the design and implementation of self-care educational efforts may be essential to establish this balance.

A host of questions related to the legal aspects of self-care will inevitably arise. Broadly, these will revolve around the modification or extension of concepts of medico-legal responsibilities. At what points, with what safeguards, and through what changes in the law can physician responsibility be appropriately transferred to laypersons? What would such a transfer then imply in terms of a reorganization of service-delivery systems, changes in needed personnel and their training? Given that self-care is a civil right of laypersons with relatively few de jure restraints and assuming that lay interest in expanding self-care continues, then this question arises: what are the criteria that define the effective limits of self-care and its corollary, the effective limits of professional medical care? As noted earlier, self-care is by and large unacknowledged in the legal literature. Statutes cover the practice of medicine, surgery, nursing, dentistry, pharmacy, etc., from the standpoint of the performance of those acts for compensation, gain, or reward, received or expected. This situation prevails in the countries represented at the Copenhagen Symposium. But there are, of course, de facto prohibitions which, although not possessing the force of law, undoubtedly would affect the public's interest and willingness to undertake to learn and apply certain procedures. One can anticipate court tests, as occurred in California recently in the case of a woman charged with the medicinal application of yogurt to another woman. Those who engage in self-care education must be made aware of such possible conflicts. Perhaps a more immediate and substantial issue is the possibility of professionals assuming de jure constraints, causing them to limit their educational efforts with laypersons to health procedures which do not impinge upon traditional medical functions.

It should be emphasized that interest in self-care extends beyond that of physicians or other direct providers. Administrators, policy-makers, governmental and private funding agencies all have great interest in developments which influence innovations in health care delivery. Potentially, policy-makers and administrators will be significant factors in the encouragement or inhibition of the growing self-care movement. For this reason, the organizers of the Copenhagen Symposium included among its participants some experienced health administrators, whose views and personal knowledge of the conditions and processes of policy change raised additional issues of implementation.

For health administrators, the questions are predominantly tactical and practical ones; for example, the nature of incentives and procedures that might encourage the assumption of self-care responsibilities by the population; and, correspondingly, the optimal modes of bringing about changes or transfers of functions by health professionals. How to implement such massive, structural changes, how to best influence and condition the correspondingly necessary alterations in public and professional attitudes clearly will be issues for both educators and policy-makers.

The steady growth of self-care as a social movement also raises some issues of broad political significance. Especially in the United States, where much political effort has been mobilized for the expansion and improvement of health delivery, promotion of self-care has been questioned as diversionary and disruptive of these goals. Some political strategists believe that "self-help" or "self-care" may play into the hands of those who would limit movements for more equitable and higher quality health services under public provision, thus diminishing professional and public responsibility.

This concern may indeed have some surface plausibility, but to us it rests upon a misunderstanding of the true nature and potential of self-care. Self-care is corollary to professional care; it is a primary and essential element in health care, and its strengthening can result only in increasing the efficacy of the professional resource by reducing iatrogenesis and enhancing role precision. However, professionals, health systems, planners, and government bodies may have to modify many elements of their philosophy, structures, policies, and procedures to adapt to self-care. That new combinations and distributions of functions would subsequently occur was a strongly expressed view of several participants.

Nevertheless, this shift of emphasis would in no way imply a lessening of needed *total* health resources, but in many respects an increase of certain kinds—e.g., educational and instructional resources. Nor can the economic consequences of enhanced self-care be assessed at this point, in view of many uncertainties associated with consumer needs and effective demand.

We do not presume to make any political judgment, but it is of interest to note that self-care also has attracted as great interest in countries, such as the United Kingdom and Denmark, which have national health systems, as in the United States, which does not. Strengthening self-care, therefore, seems to represent a basic thrust toward a more adequate, more accessible, more dignified, and possibly more effective mode of using health resources, irrespective of the particular health delivery or financing system or, for that matter, political environment.

If popular competence in self-care is to be enhanced through educational modalities, decisions about the deployment and the types of professional workers needed in the new delivery structures will, of course, be pertinent. A related and key issue concerns the nature of the medical and other professional education needed to reflect the changing balance between professional and lay health care functions. As self-care emerges, curricula in health professional education would have to reflect new objectives and methods coordinate with achieving a "partnership attitude" in health practitioners and the *skills* involved in passing along diagnostic and treatment strategies appropriate to self-care. This might require new forces of joint lay-professional learning at all levels. These would serve to diminish the counterproductive aspects of the presently dissociating and alienating separation between professional and lay education in health.

From these diverse perspectives, a major issue emerges with regard to how concepts of the appropriate balance or mixture between professional and lay activity in health care will be formulated. As has been indicated earlier, current definitions of health and illness, the criteria for the attribution of a state of illness in an individual, have been assumed to be exclusively in the domain of professional judgment. If a change occurs in the involvement of lay persons in their own health care, including the elements of symptom perception, self-diagnosis, self-medication, and other autotherapies, then it seems clear that definition, even the certification of illness states, also will probably involve important inputs from laypersons. Some examples of informal tendencies along this line have been emerging from the experience of self-help groups, as previously described. Whatever else might be said of these groups, their success in dealing with certain addictions or in heightening motivation toward recovery and rehabilitation for chronically, physically disabled persons makes it certain that a re-evaluation of the professional's monopolistic claims to knowledge will be one consequence of the growth of self-care.

Ethical Issues

Many of the ethical issues surrounding the concept of self-care are corollary to its primary effect: the sharing of power through the redistribution of technical skills and the strengthening of lay initiatives in decision-making. A number of derivative concerns were expressed at the Copenhagen meeting: What about damage (i.e., malpractice)? What are the risks of false positives and false negatives, of over-medication, etc.? Is society prepared to trade off some avoidable damage against the presumed health, social-psychological, and economic benefits of self-care?

Then, there is concern about "imposing" self-care on society as a whole. Perhaps some members of the population would *prefer* to remain passive and dependent. Should self-care be specifically aimed at present sub-populations, including high-risk groups such as inappropriate over-users of professional services, or should it be generally promoted?

While the Copenhagen Symposium concluded with no explicit concensus on either the ethics or strategy of targeting self-care education, there was a clear and continuous theme throughout discussions which emphasized the primacy of benefits to the layperson (medical, social, economic) over organizational or administrative benefits if and when these are not of apparent and immediate *mutual* benefit. In effect, several discussants were concerned that self-care not be promoted as a device to manipulate the consumer of health services to fit the exigencies or convenience of the provider system. The airing of this issue served to clarify and reiterate the view that self-care as it is now and as it could be further developed is an option—that additional degree of freedom to choose from among several courses of action—that action which is in the laypersons' best interest as they see it.

On the other side of the coin is the issue of inducing or prolonging patient dependency, and the ethic of denying patients the opportunity to achieve greater self-determination. This broad issue encompasses several more specific ones: obligation to inform patients of their diagnosis, of treatment options, and prognosis, and the sharing of medical record with the patient as a civil right as well as a sound medical practice. What, if any, are the justifiable grounds for *not* maximizing patient self-determination?

The historic defenses for maintaining patient passivity (to achieve greater compliance), withholding information on diagnosis and treatment (to eliminate patient confusion: i.e., "a little knowledge is a dangerous thing"), or obfuscating prognosis (to reduce patient anxiety) are being challenged by consumer advocacy groups and in the popular literature. Some recent titles (*How to Choose and Use Your Doctor, Managing Your Doctor, How to Help Your Doctor Help You,* and *Talk Back to Your Doctor*)[7] are representative of a popular interest in enhancing effective patient participation in the clinical encounter.

The Symposium participants reflected some of the ambivalence which often accompanies discussion of radical change in the doctor-patient relationship, particularly when such deeply rooted traditions as the medical record are being discussed. Concern for possible misuse, misunderstanding, and breaching confidentiality suggests the importance placed on these artifacts of practice as symbolic and operating factors in the phenomenon called "trust" or "faith." The mystique of medicine as *content* of practice and the associated placebo strategies are well known. The visit to the doctor itself, as a source of validation for illness, must be considered in anticipating the impact of self-care and self-determination. Here the sense of argument was not for holding rigidly to the position of doctor-centered control, but to consider the implications of self-care for diminishing the therapeutic (as well as iatrogenic) contributions of trust and validation in care. There may well be, as several participants noted, a change in the *basis* of trust; less unilateral, less diffuse; more reflective of a state of interdependence rather than either dependence or independence.

Quality Assurance and Cost Effectiveness

Self-care as it is now practiced is subject to empirical testing, although the criteria of effectiveness may not always coincide with professional criteria. Professional evaluations of the efficacy of self-care practices now run the gamut from charges of dangerous and ineffectual empiricism, to the view that they are generally harmless, often appropriate, and that they indeed make it possible to save health care systems, especially primary care, from being swamped. The research of Poul Pedersen of Denmark and John Fry of Britain gives support to the latter and more positive assessments.

Medical experience in general indicates that most common illness is self-limiting and is rarely life-threatening. This fact renders appropriate a greater attention to and use of self-care modalities.

It is by no means certain, however, that the ideal of a totally self-care competent society would result in overall cost reduction. Although one could theorize that high levels of self-care competence would impact on both costs to individuals and on the medical-economic monopolies, there is no solid basis for predicting how economic benefits would be redistributed among consumers and the several components of the medical-industrial complex. Discussion of the economics of self-care was largely speculative, leading toward recommendations for national and cross-national economic impact studies reflecting a balanced effort between clinically oriented cost-benefit research and more macro analyses of systems impacts and demographic impacts.

That self-care development programs require and should have the most searching and vigorous empirical investigation is self-evident. Detailed discussion of the whats, hows, and whys of such studies occupied much of the Copenhagen meeting and will be reviewed in the next chapter.

References

[1] Lester Breslow, "Basic Foundations of Personal Health Care," in Maxcy-Rosenau, *Preventive Medicine and Public Health* (10th ed.), (New York: Appleton-Century Crofts, 1973), pp. 633–676.

[2] *Ibid.*

[3] Thomas H. Holmes, "Multi-Discipline Studies in Tuberculosis," in Sparer (ed.), *Personality, Stress and Tuberculosis* (New York: International Universities Press, 1956), pp. 65–146.

[4] Lawrence E. Hinkle and Norman Plummer, "Life Stress and Industrial Absenteeism," *Industrial Medicine and Surgery* 21 (August 1952), pp. 365–375.

[5] H. Mahler, "Health—A Demystification of Medical Technology," *Lancet* (November 1, 1975), pp. 829–833.

[6] See, for example, Alfred H. Katz and Eugene I. Bender, *The Strength in Us: Self-Help Groups in the Modern World* (New York: Franklin Watts, 1976).

[7] See "Self-Care in Health" Annotated Bibliography (Consumer-Provider Relationships).

CHAPTER V

Research Challenges in Self-Care

It is apparent that at the present time there are only meager data regarding the practices of self-care; the problems it addresses or causes; and the nature of its technical, social, political, and organizational effects. There is no adequate thesaurus or retrieval system to define or set forth the nature, magnitude, or any more limited aspect of self-care, except on a very restricted, parochial basis.[1] No international classification of self-care practices is available.

These lacks suggest that self-care is generally taken for granted as an element in health care. It is viewed largely as a marginal phenomenon, perhaps of interest to anthropologists, but receives only peripheral attention as a factor in health care delivery. Participants at the Copenhagen Symposium agreed that studies of the lay component in primary care, in contrast to studies of the professional component, were almost totally lacking in research and rarely considered in health planning. These reasons alone give prima facie justification to undertaking descriptive, empirical, and analytic research. The present data from clinical impressions, practice-based studies, and survey research serve to underscore the need to give high priority to systematic study of self-care. Several Symposium participants felt that as we are now proceeding to understand the limits of the professional health resource, so a corollary systematic examination of self-care should be begun.

A commitment to self-care research should not demand philosophical allegiance of investigators to its promotion or discredit. Discussions in Copenhagen were helpful in illuminating this point. It was often difficult to ignore a considerable emotional factor, both latent and expressed, on the subject of self-care. Several Symposium participants raised the issue of objectivity in research and the potential for bias and prejudicial effects in this politically sensitive area. One commented:

> We must be very careful not to take out our frustration on the existing medical establishment whose help will be needed in any improvement . . . Change must be based on substantive evaluation. Medicine is a support system for society. We must be sure to understand the values of the potential consumers before we change what medicine offers society.

This concern in part derives from the popular base of interest in self-care and the exaggerated effects that could ensue from the misinterpretation of fragmentary research. More important, these cautions reflect an awareness that self-care research and demonstration will have to address such sensitive issues as the efficacy of present primary care technology, the substitutive potentials in primary care of lay skills, and the implications of self-care for reducing iatrogenic effects and improving professional services. These topics lie at the interface of established values and beliefs of professionals as well as of laypersons. It was hoped that self-care research could be conducted with objectivity, without prejudgment of what is or what should be.

These considerations emphasize that scientific inquiry is never a rapid or a simple process. It requires painstaking intellectual labor throughout all its stages, from initial observation/description, problem definition/formulation, hypothesis-generation, data gathering and analysis, evaluation of hypotheses in the light of data, to final assessment of significance.

A Theoretical Framework for Self-Care Research

Some Copenhagen participants noted that there is no theoretical framework for looking at self-care. Others held the contrary view: that there is, in fact, a rich literature of theories, postulates, and hypotheses relevant to self-care. However, these have not been integrated into a global rationalization, a mapping of determinants of self-care behavior, or self-care as an independent variable influencing health status and the use of organized health resources. An ordered assemblage of complementary theories coupled with a sorting of descriptive and experimental documentation would provide a useful baseline for planning a comprehensive, articulated research strategy. One might begin by organizing the extant theory and research in relation to the classical categories of health maintenance behavior, risk-reducing behavior, illness behavior, sick role behavior, rehabilitation behavior, and chronic care behavior. This would provide a descriptive listing from which gaps and incongruities in theory and research relevant to self-care could be identified.

Further, such an analysis might reveal assumptive biases which would result in failures to test the full range of behavioral effects. An example of possible bias is research on delay in seeking medical care. The usual assumption of research on this phenomenon is that delay is inappropriate and needs to be studied to reduce or eliminate it. A less judgmental approach to research on delay would focus on the quality of the decision-making process as the key variable. The consequences of decisions would be examined in terms of outcomes which allow for the probabilities of positive, non-significant, and negative effects as measured against both patient and professional criteria.

Getting the theoretical house in order is an ambitious undertaking for any aspect of socio-medical research. As has been noted earlier, self-care presents unique problems. Self-care practices pervade in the broader system of social behavior and, therefore, are most difficult to isolate in pristine theoretical terms. Hence, initial research strategies may have to restrict theoretical development to a definition of self-care which can account for those behaviors a *given culture* interprets as purposeful self-interventions with specific expectations of health promotion, illness prevention, treatment, restoration, and iatrogenic control. The key ingredient in building self-care theory is reliance on the culturally determined behavioral categories, with professionally derived categories being viewed as supplementary, not subordinate. The integrity of self-care theory is its ability to predict behavior as a function of lay, professional, and institutional attributes and it must emerge, therefore, as a synthesis of perspectives.

Researchable Issues

The Symposium encompassed many diverse views and suggestions concerning pertinent approaches to one or more of the *stages* of self-care research. In the interests of systematization, but without claim to comprehensiveness, this great variety of views, suggestions, insights, and possible hypotheses have been organized and will be discussed under four main headings: Social Studies; Clinical and Educational Studies in Self-Care; Studies Relating to Professional Interest in Self-Care; and Policy Studies: Economic and Organizational.

The major thrust of the Symposium lay in this attempt to formulate researchable issues. Many participant comments, not specifically directed toward research issues, were nevertheless pertinent to the preliminary phases in research of problem definition, problem formulation, and hypothesis development. Discussion also centered on description and taxonomical concerns, i.e., blocking in the contours of self-care, describing its parameters, refining its definition, indicating its conceptual links and relationships with other components of the health care process. The sections that follow delineate some research questions and possibilities that evolved, grouped according to the above fourfold typology.

I. Social Studies

In the field of social phenomena, historical, cultural, and psychological forces are enormously important. Each society may be said to construct its own health system according to these three kinds of idiosyncratic factors. Description and specification of the present varieties of self-care, in their recent historical development as well as in their specific current manifestations, is required as a first phase in descriptive research.

Cultural influences might include the diverse effects of political and religious ideologies, popular beliefs and attitudes, as they affect a particular culture's views of health in general, and self-care in health in particular. These are basic to an understanding of the pertinence of new self-care efforts in health, and the probability of their adoption and diffusion in any particular setting.

Historical and social perspectives are likewise essential to an informed view of current manifestations of self-care. Understanding can ensue only as the drive to self-care is seen as arising today from the many successes of modern medicine and public health, not merely as a reaction to their failures and deficiencies. A comprehensive account of the development in various societies of health care as a social institution would indicate that self-care today is not merely a harking-back to a pre-scientific period of folk beliefs, but builds upon and employs scientific knowledge. Self-care presupposes *an active and educated public,* active on their own behalf, and educated through a variety of formal and informal channels, in the application of effective health care practices.

A related question of historical and social importance is the role of interest groups. It is predictable that any meeting held to discuss self-care at this time of renewed interest in the phenomenon will express curiosity about the question of "why now?" The Copenhagen Symposium brought together an ad hoc group of health practitioners, administrators, and social scientists who, as individuals, had professional involvement or interest in self-care. Yet the early part of the Symposium was dominated by discussion intended to clarify the *causes* of current interest in self-care, the *sources* or loci of mobilized interest, and the legitimacy of self-care as a coherent social innovation, transcending mere fad or fantasy. Participants' experiences with, and their varied perspectives on self-care stimulated concern with questions related to cross-national interest in self-care. This interest does not seem to flow from the usual progression of extensive research, or from national health policy or program commitments. In a real sense, the conferees asked for research that would remove or confirm doubts about the wisdom of mounting serious professional and academic investments in self-care development. A contribution to this decision would be an understanding of the basis of the present organized interest in self-care.

In this connection, the principal questions posed were: What are the characteristics, motivation, and expectations of individuals and groups engaged in self-care developments? To whom are their efforts addressed and with what objectives and methods? What linkages exist with social organizations and a health care system? Are there channels for communication among self-care interest groups? What factors influence their growth, viability, and maintenance? Answers to these questions would permit assessment of the realities of self-care as a contemporary health, social, and political phenomenon and help clarify the appropriate corollary role of professional and scholarly resources. Other periods of history offer evidence of lay interest in incorporating scientific or professional knowledge and technology as a supplement to, or substitute for, indigenous self-care practices in health. At present, it was noted that there is a plethora of treatises and texts for the instruction of nonprofessional primary care givers within the family context. One can readily trace the tradition and evolution of lay self-care literature, but it would be hazardous to attempt to deduce the social, medical, and cultural forces which influenced both the character of the advice sought and the advice given. At best there is historical evidence that interest in self-care has a "market-place" significance.

Examination of the self-care literature would offer only marginal clues as to the intensity, extent, and specificity of *lay* initiatives in promoting self-care. Even if a retrospective study of lay initiatives in self-care could be accomplished technically, any interpretation of findings as relevant to the very recent past and to the present would have to account for extraordinary shifts in the context and social significance of health and disease. This would have to include the concepts of specialization and professionalism. A more feasible approach appears to be one which emphasizes recent history of current practices and provides for prospective, continuous monitoring. The cross-national perspective would add dimensions of cultural, social-philosophical, and political variations in conformity with the international perspective recommended by the Symposium for other aspects of self-care research.

Several variables were identified as important in influencing lay interest in self-care. It was assumed that, as the genesis of self-care interest reflects many factors, these variables must be studied through an epidemiologic design. Of special interest are the following questions:

1. What is the relationship between the increased prevalence of chronic disease and the demand for self-care skills?

2. Are rising levels of educational attainment in a population associated with increased demand for self-care skills?

3. Does the presence or absence of "anti-technology" and "anti-authority" sentiments bear a relationship to a population's interest in (a) self-care skills, and (b) strategies for gaining greater lay control over the professional care system?

4. Is there a relationship between the level of consumer activism in a population, and the demand for self-care?

5. What is the relationship between the level of consumer participation (community control) in health care systems and citizen demand for self-care skills?

6. What influence has the growth of the physician extender concept and other non-physician models had on public perspectives on self-care?

7. How do the de-mystification of medical knowledge, public skepticism about medicine's effectiveness, and cynicism about physicians' economic motives affect the demand for self-care?

8. Is there a relationship between the general economic climate and demand for self-care skills?

9. In what ways are popular interests in alternative health care methods, e.g., meditation, healing, biofeedback, linked to interest in self-care?

10. What impact does increased specialization and the concomitant decrease in primary care resources have on demand for self-care skills?

Clearly, other aspects of developing national experiences (e.g., National Health Insurance in the United States; reorganization of the Danish social welfare system in 1971) should be considered in their impact on levels of popular interest in self-care.

II. Clinical and Educational Studies in Self-Care

A. Criteria for self-care skills As noted earlier, many kinds of self-care have been practiced, with wide historical and cultural variation. Some observers believe that most health care is in fact self-care. However, opinions differ on how much of it involves symptomatic relief or treatment of minor non-disabling illness on the one hand, or treatment of disabling illness and self-intervention in life-threatening episodes on the other. A few studies in Great Britain and the United States suggest that the level of non-medically attended illness and injury is sufficiently high to show a wide range of self-care practices, beyond the mere relief of symptoms and care of minor illnesses and injuries. The few available studies concerning the relevance and efficacy of extant self-care practices offer some evidence that the self-care interventions which preceded professional treatment were quite appropriate. Such studies, helpful as pioneering efforts, now must be followed by more broadly based population surveys of the extent of self-care practices, along with sample studies of particular practices as they affect care outcomes. The United States National Health Survey, with an in-depth clinical review of a sub-sample of the study population, may be a useful model for such studies.

As additions to the existing armamentarium of self-care skills are considered, a new set of issues and research requirements arises. The central reality must be faced that the decision to transfer clinical skills from practitioner to layperson is by no means an exclusive decision of the professional. Indeed, recently such transfers have been largely based on lay initiatives, and the influences of popular literature. The lay self-care movement must not and will not be subject to domination by professionals through their unilateral decisions about what clinical skills will be transferred to the laity, or how this will occur. This does not suggest a merely passive role for the professions. On the contrary, given an interest in developing a more medically competent citizenry, the health professional can undertake: (1) to carefully assess established clinical practices (preventive through rehabilitative) for their essential worth; and (2) to establish technical criteria for the selection of clinical skills appropriate for transfer. Let us take a closer look at these tasks.

During an intense discussion of the skill transfer issue, one general medical practitioner raised the question of how secure we were in our belief in the effectiveness of the primary care skills in professional practice. There was mounting concern (and some evidence), he observed, that some of the traditional procedures may at best be used for their placebo effect and at worst are wasteful of time and money or even injurious to the patient. Furthermore, some practices may contribute inordinately to the creation or prolongation of patient dependency. Elaboration of this and similar comments heightened emphasis on the responsibility of professionals interested in self-care development to undertake an objective self-appraisal of primary care procedures.

Evaluation of this kind is both practicable and compatible with the routines of medical practice. Basic to the evaluative procedure is the record-keeping system, and its utility in the correlation of problems, procedures, and outcome notes. Based on their own experience, several practitioners at Copenhagen confirmed the potential for such mini-research and its multiple benefits, clinical and epidemiologic. Data protocols, recording, and retrieval systems may be adopted from those designed by practitioners. The application of a problem-oriented record system[2] could add a useful framework for procedural audits of the type required for decisions about skill transfers as well as for appraisal of the contribution of the patients' already established self-care skills. A companion record system[3] maintained by the patient may be a valuable corollary resource in the latter regard. It could emphasize patients' recording of self-initiated care procedures relating to conditions not seen by the practitioner, and notations on the effectiveness of professional procedures applying patient-oriented criteria.

These thoughts suggest the need to supplement practitioner observations with a broader data base which reflects a wide range of clinical experience and patient populations. Resultant data are requisites to more universal tests of validity and reliability.

Having established the efficacy of a clinical procedure, there remains the matter of the appropriateness of the transfer procedure from the standpoint of its technology. The criteria that might apply are the central issues here; both the questions posed and the answers given may be deceptively simple. For example, the common initial reaction is that the transferred procedure should not be "dangerous." But it is obvious that the concept of danger is relative and contingent. What may be dangerous depends on the operator's competence, the design of the instrumentation, the clarity and fail-safe value of the procedural protocol, and upon attributes of the procedure, process, and operator. Furthermore, time is also a factor that may increase or diminish competence. In addition, there is the social environment and the nature of its contributing support to the person or family undertaking a procedure. Thus, the notion of "danger" has to be assessed according to specific circumstances. "Danger" as an isolated possibility, independent of other attributes, is difficult to assess. One must, for example, also take into account the differences in the potential for clinical iatrogenesis of self-care as well as both the clinical and social iatrogenesis consequential to procedures professionally performed.

Other criteria for the process of technical decision-making in transferring certain functions to lay people have similar difficulties, e.g., frequency of use. A distinction must clearly be made between how many times a procedure is called upon, i.e., its intensivity, and the duration of its use, i.e., its extensivity. A family care-giver may frequently use skills in diagnosing and treating childhood diseases, but only during one period of the family life cycle. Some disease-specific procedures are useful only at a given stage of morbidity. Thus, frequency as a criterion requires a context.

The availability of technical equipment, the educational costs of training the layperson to use complex technology, and the requirements for continuing education of the layperson are also criteria frequently mentioned. Again a variety of contingencies clusters around each. Technology undergoes rapid development and simplification—witness the blood pressure cuff and dialysis. The more imaginative use and greater availability of mass communication media, such as two-way telecommunications in continuing education of practitioners, offer new possibilities for lay access to continuing education resources.

From these considerations, the research task in technical criteria-setting would seem to require a systems approach, which allows for criteria contingencies, as noted, and further posits the interaction of criteria. Based on this assumption, the goal of technical criteria-setting would be to develop a matrix of data relevant to a given procedure, sufficiently simple in design to permit a "balance sheet" decision-making process to occur. The matrix would be multi-dimensional with axes and surfaces which calibrate characteristics of the procedure (e.g., complexity, time/money costs), the client (e.g., interest, competence, supportive resources, intensivity/extensivity of use), and the practitioner-educator (e.g., teaching capabilities, relationship with client).

Developing such a decision-making model is clearly a long-range task, demanding inputs from several disciplines as well as continuing advice from clinicians. It would serve as a guiding device for practitioners and health service planners, offering a framework for decision-making regarding self-care skill transfer—not pre- or proscribing the practitioner's technical decisions. Further, the focus of the decision-making process is not solely in terms of a disease category, but on self-care functions or procedures which may prove to have more general educational benefits, both preventive and curative. These would be appropriate for community as well as patient education.

B. Developing self-care education strategies Some intermediate level studies may be identified which could contribute to criteria-setting as well as the design of lay self-care education strategies. Foremost among these is the need to examine the present and potential of self-care functions relevant to specific disease states (e.g., hypertension, diabetes), where the self-care benefits seem particularly great. Similarly, research priority might be given to broader types of health problems or morbid conditions that may be especially susceptible to self-care modalities. Symposium participants suggested as appropriate target populations the physically disabled, children and adolescents, and the elderly.

Such studies should be designed within the accepted parameters of clinical trials, where self-care skill competence, either as a result of educational efforts or spontaneous practices initiated by the patient, can be assessed by specified clinical and social outcomes. Evaluation of self-care should transcend its impact on the disease state by involving measures of its effects on the patient-physician relationship. In this aspect of self-care research, in addition to an analysis of patient satisfaction,[4] it is also relevant to observe differences in the patient's orientation to the physician; namely, the degree of mutuality or dominance in the relationship.[5] Independent observations of the patient's self-confidence, using the concept of locus of control, would be of signal relevance.[6]

Corollary to perceived differences in patient status is the reaction of the professional in interaction with the self-care active patient. Using a "double blind" research design, it should be possible to observe the impact of substitution of roles and other aspects of patient control on the professional's behavior. Such data could be useful in designing educational experiences for health professionals aimed at helping them anticipate and derive satisfaction from work with patients who are active and competent participants in their own care.

C. Clinical and descriptive studies of self-care in the community setting The preceding discussion of technical criteria-setting and the development of outcome measures reflects the Symposium's concern that professional interventions in self-care should not embody or exacerbate any risks in health care. Micro-level studies of the kind described would help clarify and delimit the professional's role in self-care development. Within the terms of their perspectives it would also offer an agenda for self-care education of the community.

Several community self-care education "clinical trials" were proposed, using independent variables ranging from education for general health-promoting skills, to specific disease treatment skills. It was suggested that self-care field experiments be undertaken in situations which have socio-political homogeneity; that is in communities formed by a common identity of shared interests, needs, or concerns. This strategy would allow for more precision and relevance in the selection of educational inputs, increase the likelihood of a more effective diffusion of practices, and make longitudinal evaluations of outcome more feasible. Outcome measures would reflect aggregated health and social changes as a consequence of accelerated self-care education. This would involve use of both established health indicators (e.g., disease incidence and prevalence) and resource-consumption indicators. Analyses of data would reveal variations among specific population groups, such as socioeconomic, racial, ethnic, sex, age-specific.

While accepting the need and utility of such studies of professionally determined outcome measures, there is an equally important need to evaluate some of the unique aspects of self-care. These aspects would include the determinants of lay capability and confidence in health decision-making in self-care, and resulting effects on levels of clinical and social iatrogenesis. Evaluation of these aspects of self-care will require significant lay inputs concerning what to observe and on the methods of observation. Design of a self-care educational research plan must also reflect awareness that new self-care inputs are not being entered on a tabula rasa. An established set of beliefs, techniques, and preferences in health already exists for each individual and group. The aim of self-care education is to offer additional technology and options within the context of present health behaviors. Thus, the descriptive data base required would entail knowledge of extant self-care practices and lay attitudes about desirable changes in them.

The interpretation of changes in behavior should reflect the differing goals of self-care education, as compared with conventional health education, which seeks to modify behavior mainly in the direction of professionally valued outcomes. Not only should self-care programs be evaluated in terms of morbidity or the use of services, but changes studied of effects on the quality of lay risk-taking decisions, and the effects of lay management of health care transactions. These considerations further reflect the need to set aside conventional biases in research on health behavior change. The question of resistance to change, for example, may not merely be one of lay resistance to changes professionals seek, but also one of professional resistance to changes sought by the layperson.

The term self-care directs attention to individual behavior and in that sense fails to capture the reality of its social dimension. Individuals both give and receive care and support, of either a supplementary or a substitutive type. The family as a health care environment has been well described,[7] but a variety of other social institutions may offer comparable or complementary health care support to their members (e.g., peer groups, work place relations). The concept of the lay health care support system in self-care includes the lay referral system. However, the aspect of the lay health care process of central interest is the care function itself—diagnosis, treatment, and assistance in managing the professional care resource. Investigation concerning the social dimensions of self-care must take into account the variations in social organization among different cultures and social groups. Categories of inquiry with regard to the index care-giver might include the following:

- Socio-demographic characteristics of the lay care-giver
- Social relationship of the lay care-giver *vis-à-vis* the recipients of care
- Source of ascribed special competence of care-giver
- Reasons and circumstances for initiating care-giving
- Range of care-giving behaviors
- Reciprocity between index care-giver and recipient(s)
- Time, duration, continuity, frequency of care provided
- Nature of gratification and performance reinforcement
- Economic consequences of the care given

Of special interest is the larger social-cultural environment's effect upon the extent and character of self-care as an "other-oriented" activity.

D. Evaluation of self-care education programs and available educational materials Preparations for the Symposium and information presented by participants gave an impression of a small but growing number of self-care educational programs designed for specific lay groups (e.g., rural communities, middle-class adults, inner-city poor, women's groups). There were, however, only modest data available on program evaluation and what was available appeared fragmentary. The reasons for this are numerous: the relative newness of the programs; the spontaneity of their emergence; the lack of evaluative expertise in the sponsoring groups; the belief that the benefits were self-evident; the costs of careful evaluation; and the lack of appropriate evaluative measures.

At the same time, there has been a burgeoning self-care oriented literature, some emanating from the experience of formal educational programs. These materials include algorithms, protocols, signs-symptoms-treatment regimens, preventive information, chronic disease management, and strategies for controlling the iatrogenic effects of professional care.[8] They constitute a torrent of materials whose appeal, benefits, or shortcomings are generally unknown. What and whose criteria of judgment should be applied is a question second only to that of the social ethic within which social control might be applied. The Symposium gave no suggestion of censorship, but a positive concern that the layperson as client or citizen have increasing access to high quality, current information and technology. These materials, it was agreed, should be made more accessible and relevant to the world community.

The Symposium discussion emphasized the importance of beginning cross-cultural evaluations of self-care education programs and materials. Recognizing the importance of maintaining relevance of content and the unique character of each client group, comparative analyses would not be concerned with standard outcomes but rather with changes relevant to the expectations of particular client groups.[9] In addition, there are opportunities to study variations in the medical practice cultures as expressed in algorithms and protocol design where they are in use.

E. Self-care education of school-age children There was a generally acknowledged assumption among many Symposium participants that the most profound and pervasive potential for self-care development resides in the education of children. While self-care skills can be learned virtually at any age, the attitudes and perspectives which emerge regarding personal initiative in health decisions and self-control in health care are often influenced negatively by the socialization process. School health education, where available, has by and large perpetuated a view of health care which suppresses or severely limits the growth of values and beliefs that the individual is competent as the primary source of health maintenance. Health "facts" are presented to children as secure and immutable; health professionals as possessing skills fixed and demarcated from those available to laypersons. "Folk medicine" or home remedies and indigenous health customs are often denigrated as quaint, ineffective, and sometimes dangerous.

While a few noteworthy exceptions exist[10] these are scattered examples and hardly constitute a force for change. Yet childhood is probably where we should begin; with exemplary models and the testing of innovative approaches aimed at strengthening the child's self-perception as a competent health decision-maker, capable of increasing self-care skills within the limits of interests and ability.

The framework for self-care education in schools requires refinement of content, methods, sequencing, and evaluation. Beyond the pro forma tasks of development, there are unique aspects to school self-care education which need to be studied. Among the most difficult is the matter of linkage between the self-care educated child, the child's family, and the community of health resources. School programs in self-care will not flourish in a vacuum. A supportive cadre of adult care-givers as well as understanding of the goals of the program are essential to ensure control over mixed cultural messages.

We may conclude that there would be exciting challenges in experimenting with and evaluating various approaches to self-care education for the school-age child. An international symposium devoted to this subject could help set an agenda for development and a basis for cooperative exchange.

III. Studies Relating to Professional Interest in Self-Care

The thrust of the Copenhagen Symposium and all the discussions of this volume suggest that self-care in health is a potential or nascent social movement in the highly developed industrial society. However, it is far from the stage of widespread acceptance or incorporation in the professional health care system, even in those settings in which the greatest amount of experimentation has occurred. As much of our previous material has implied, acceptance and wider use of self-care may be accelerated through the active contributions of health practitioners, policy-makers, health planners, and administrators. Dissemination and testing of educational strategies aimed at these groups would be particularly important in increasing understanding of self-care's actual and potential effects, and in reducing misconceptions. Professional involvement in the development of self-care need not lead inevitably to professional domination. Keeping health professionals "in the dark" is not a secure preventive. The only guarantee for a balanced development resides in the growth of lay awareness of options and lay competence to pursue them.

The point at issue seems to be effective educational change, not the testing of strategies to persuade professionals on the basis of belief or polemic. Recognition of the many current data deficits in self-care suggest the need for an approach to professional education which incorporates self-care research into the teaching armory. Self-care research, jointly undertaken by faculty and students, could achieve high levels of credibility and predispose toward the application of relevant concepts and skills in practice.

Effective education in the practicing professions requires an interrelated system of theory building and opportunities to apply theory in practice. Building practitioner skills in self-care is no exception. In self-care the challenge lies in changing the practitioner and "client" expectations of the roles of the practitioner as active healer and the client as passive recipient. In such a change the sources of the professional's gratifications would shift from the practitioner's accomplishments to the "client's" accomplishments. Educational trials could test differences in the practitioner's teaching effectiveness and attitudes as these shift to an emphasis on self-care instruction in various settings. Such educational trials would also have to look at client reactions and learning as part of the evaluation.

A third component of an educational strategy aimed at students in the health professions would focus attention on concepts and theories which provide perspectives on the role of the health professions and the effects of professionalization in relation to the students' own experience. Such insights should contribute toward an understanding of popular activism in health care, and of the benefits of less dependent client-practitioner relationships. Educational efforts in this area should not be limited to didactic approaches. Recent teaching of social science concepts to health professionals has used practical or clinical activities to demonstrate theoretical points; accounts are widely available in the literature.[11]

Finally, with regard to education in self-care for health professional students, the impact of the total educational environment must be recognized. Suggestions for global changes in the scope of professional health education were beyond the charge of the Copenhagen Symposium, but certain aspects of health professional education are particularly germane to the goals of a self-care curriculum. Overcoming the traditional isolation of health professional schools from other elements of higher education is important to the effective development of a self-care orientation for their students. It would be feasible to offer selected non-health profession students an opportunity to participate with health student colleagues in courses and experiences where the central focus is on conceptual issues of the health professions in society. Such a "civilian presence" could provide a reality-testing situation of benefit to both types of student. Experimental trials at this level may generate wider innovations in the same direction.

Up to this point we have dealt with testing educational innovations in the process of formal education in the health professions. In the long run such investments might yield more substantial returns than comparable levels of effort among practicing health professionals. Perhaps the most feasible strategy is to select practice situations where external constraints to change are fewer and internal incentives are greatest. In countries with national health systems or universal health insurance, the opportunities for stimulating interest in practitioner involvement in self-care seem more hopeful. In the United States, prepaid group practices (e.g., Health Maintenance Organizations) with built-in incentives for resource use control and preventive practice seem to be appropriate environments for experimental efforts in self-care. Furthermore, such settings offer opportunity for continuous educational programs for clients and some greater likelihood of team programs. The development of self-care programs in the United States has been actively pursued by professionals in group, prepaid, hospital- or clinic-based practices. In such settings beginnings can be made to design and test self-care modalities, which would then become available to the wider community of health practitioners. Several models of self-care education might be tested as to procedures (content, clients, methods, duration) and outreach techniques (community sponsorship, fellowships, use of key influentials to attract participation).

Relevant application of innovation-diffusion theory[12,13] might offer additional insights on the more general acceptability of self-care education functions to community practitioners. Such a strategy takes into account the professional communications network, and its influence on collegial decision-making. Imaginative application of social theory in this regard could prove of singular value.

Beyond such program strategies, the possibility of designing and testing specific client-oriented self-care materials should also be considered. As described earlier, these materials are becoming increasingly available, and may prove useful as an intermediate device to secure practitioner confidence in self-care education, without threatening professional prerogatives. Studies could be undertaken to ascertain the impact of these materials on the practitioners in terms of changes in their self-care education perspectives and practice.

Demonstration efforts in educating health policy-makers, health planners, and administrators was given high priority by several Symposium participants, although tempered by skepticism about their prospects of success. The point of concern here centers on the political and social realities of policy-makers' roles. In contrast with health practitioners, policy-makers and administrators are accountable to multiple constituencies, often in less than harmonious accord. They are often required to make decisions on the basis of advice from others, whose interests are conflicting or not apparent, and where the decisions do not conform with the policy-maker's or administrator's personal values.

This suggests that the educational approach in the policy field must be flexible, considering the self-care ramifications of policies and planning goals, identifying key agents in the decision-making process, and becoming incorporated into that process through constituent education. The educational approach in policy is thus largely in situ, indirect, and persuasive. There are, of course, political and planning structures which may be especially accessible to and appropriate for the educational effort; note the Community Health Councils in Great Britain and Health Services Agencies in the United States.

Case study methods appear to be particularly useful in studying and evaluating both the process and outcome of strategies to communicate and effectuate self-care potentials in policy formulation and administration.

IV. Policy Studies: Economic and Organizational

A. Economic studies In the preceding sections of this chapter, we have suggested a range of descriptive and experimental studies on self-care phenomena and programs. By inference, these proposals also suggest the need to explore questions raised by self-care developments that will affect and be affected by policy and administrative decisions. Many of the latter questions relate to economics; they will require sophisticated economic research methodologies, e.g., the use of input-output outcome accounting matrices. Such studies are needed to undergird informed administrative decisions around priorities and strategies in self-care in terms of demonstrated or anticipated impacts on health status, costs, and the less tangible but salient values of consumer satisfaction, iatrogenesis (clinical/social), and democratic participation.

Some specific economic questions posed as central to self-care development are as follows:

1. What are the present costs of self-care (non-professional activities); how are these borne differentially among population groups and which population groups profit by these expenditures? Available literature on consumer costs in self-care are limited to estimates based on the consumption of products: e.g., medications (over-the-counter drugs) and certain health care products (exercise equipment, toothbrushes, first-aid materials, and the like). The costs of self-diagnosis and self-treatment (including time) are unknown. Accounting for costs will require some difficult decisions regarding the valuation of lay self-services. What should be the standard (comparable professional service costs?) and how should such a standard be weighted to reflect and correct for indirect costs?

The "cost to whom" question may be deceptively simple. A mere patient-provider framework offers a rather limited site for investigating questions of cost, since the self-provision of care frequently involves others both as support resources and beneficiaries of the self-care activity. Hence, several variations of the unit cost in self-care must be considered. Finally, some aspects of self-care embody integral components of life-style and equally serve social needs other than health (child-rearing activities, for example). How should these factors be considered in self-care cost analysis?

Methodological as well as definitional problems abound. Reporting of self-care (or any other aspect of social activity) is notoriously unreliable in terms of recall; and direct observation by external monitoring presents both tactical and ethical problems. Self-recording devices may offer some promise, but they, too, present problems of intrusion and inconvenience. Yet this area of inquiry is fundamental to studies of pertinence, both to programmatic and policy development.

An important aspect of the cost issue is the matter of who profits in the economic sense from outlays associated with self-care activities. Would significant increments in self-care activity portend major shifts in profit distribution[14] with concomitant potential for abuse? Could, in effect, a new monopoly emerge without the precedent of social regulation, thus adding another factor to burgeoning health care costs? Such questions are raised out of concern for a realistic perspective on costs and profits, given the often expressed belief that self-care practice would have a salutory effect on overall expenditures for health and reduce the profit motive (commercialization-industrialization) in health care. The potential reassignment of both costs and profits would appear worthy of monitoring.

Following the above set of questions, it might be hypothesized that self-care will significantly reduce costs specifically associated with hospitalization. Exploration of this effect of self-care would require discriminant delineations by diagnosis, patient characteristics, length of stay, and readmissions for the same complaint as well as initial admission rates. Hospital-based studies, however, would only marginally test such an hypothesis. It would also be necessary to gather data on the population at risk for hospitalization, in order to ascertain the true level of the population's exercise of the hospitalization option versus non-hospitalization options and the relationship of these decisions to levels of self-care activity, with other factors held constant. Studies should be designed for both situations of extant self-care activity (descriptive) and self-care educated populations (experimental). Studies of similar nature can be undertaken regarding the use of ambulatory care services.

2. More precision is required in isolating the particular benefits of specific self-care practices. This may become a critical area of inquiry assuming finite resources of education (or its competition with other social needs) to provide self-care skills. Which domains or processes of self-care are most cost-effective, given the costs of

training, skill maintenance costs, use frequency, implications for preventions or disability limitation, among other qualifying factors? Outcome accounting matrices for self-care practices can contribute useful data for policy determinations.

3. On the other side of the coin, what can be anticipated regarding the economic impact of self-care on health care practitioners (particularly primary care physicians) and health care institutions in countries with free market economies? The answer is relevant to one aspect of the issue of practitioner and institutional resistance to adapting practices to a self-care model, i.e., anticipated loss of income. The reality of this prospect is unknown, given the alternative possibility that, unencumbered by providing many routine or minor procedures, or by being free of many preventable complaints, the care providers are able to widen their service catchments to include more patients with complaints requiring more complex medical intervention. Monitoring of provider experience in this regard could provide data of import to health manpower planners in developing legislation regulating the production of caregivers by specialty. It is interesting to speculate how such data (in concert with other evidence of self-care's impact on health service use) might form an approach to manpower allocation and distribution based on a population's level of self-care competency. This differs from the present practice (e.g., population/physician ratios) which appears to assume standard units of professional competence and standard units of lay incompetence.

4. What economic incentives might be offered providers to encourage self-care practices and to implement self-care education programs for consumers? Interest and opportunity may not be sufficient in themselves. Educational services, when conceived as an additional services benefit, must be subject to fiscal accounting and budgeting. Health services, particularly primary care services, are labor-intensive, where use of time and personnel are the critical cost factors. It is likely, therefore, that individual and institutional providers in free-market economies will require compensation as an additional incentive. In such situations, careful cost analyses must be made, schedules established, and an accountability system worked out. This requirement undoubtedly will be the key to the enactment of governmental reimbursement legislation.

A variety of incentive schemes need to be tried in terms of both the integrity of their cost-benefit rationale[15] and their equity as perceived by the provider.

5. Health providers are, of course, only one sector of many social resources that would be involved in self-care education. Indeed, the professional health sector may be a relatively minor component in relation to the many other social institutions with potentially interested client systems. Public education is the most obvious example. Most important are the vast array of lay groups who have been a prime stimulus to the emergence and development of self-care programs. The women's self-help health collectives in the United States are examples. How society can absorb the costs of accelerated self-care development is both a question of social priorities and a question of social equity. Perhaps a more approachable question, which suggests a strategy of general support through public funds, is how existing sources of support might be made available and acceptable to self-care undertakings. The design and implementation of such a vast and sensitive undertaking must be a shared responsibility of all groups with self-care interests.

B. Studies of Health Care and Health Organization A series of hypotheses were put forward by Symposium participants as attempts to test the relationship between various characteristics of the health care system and levels of self-care interest and practice in the lay community. These hypotheses, for the most part, had a common ground: to define the mutuality of impact, to identify the linkages between the two pair "systems," and to characterize the potential of their mutual adaptability.

By and large, these hypotheses were limited to tests of the self-care effects of the layperson in the role of patient. They were grounded on the assumption that the physician is the key influence in determining the level of patient self-care activity; and further that the availability of high quality, accessible, acceptable, and continuous primary care constitutes a preferred substitute for self-care. Given a comprehensive high quality professional primary care resource, this view holds that patients' enthusiasm for self-care would diminish. It is clear that it is based on a narrowly circumscribed definition of self-care functions and potentials. But in addition to the broader perspectives of self-care development several participants believed it is also necessary to test hypotheses which apply the self-care concept in more limited terms of venue, i.e., the patient-physician dyad, and of functional definition, i.e., substitution of specific primary care skills. For such studies the following hypotheses are proposed:

1. That in a capitation fee system the physician is more likely to encourage patient self-care than would be the case in a fee-for-service system. This hypothesis assumes an influential patient-physician relationship and a more positive attitude toward self-care on the part of physicians unencumbered by concern for income loss resulting from patient self-care practices.

2. That self-care activity is greater in patient populations subject to fee-for-service than is the case for patient populations in prepaid or capitation situations. Here, in contrast to 1., above, the assumption is that the factor of direct costs of medical care to be borne by the patient would increase the patient's motivation (or necessity) to pursue self-care strategies.

3. That patient self-activity is related to the availability and accessibility of acceptable primary care options. Thus, self-care activity is likely to be greater among patients in countries where there is a multiple source primary health care system (as in Sweden and the United States) than in a single source primary health care system (as in Denmark and England).

In designing studies to test these and other hypotheses, the relationship of other aspects of health care organization to levels of patient self-care activity should be considered in their cultural context. Such studies should consider group versus solo practice; variations as a function of setting (physician's office, general hospital, ambulatory care departments, and voluntary health organizations, neighborhood health centers); and single disciplinary versus multidisciplinary care systems. Study of such organizational patterns could illuminate additional dimensions of the impact of self-care, e.g., the question of the impact of accelerated levels of self-care on the preferential use of intermediate level primary health care providers such as nurse practitioners or health aides in the instruction of patients in self-care. A companion hypothesis might be: that increasing levels of self-care competence among patients will cause primary care physicians to become less isolated and more involved with non-medical but health-related community resources.

Quality Control Studies

The Copenhagen discussions reflected a continuous concern with regard to quality control and the need to study the policy and procedural questions involved. There was a clear awareness that newly initiated and promulgated programs of self-care development must be particularly sensitive to the protection of the public regardless of their sponsorship. As soon as interference with existing levels and normative development of self-care activity occurs, it becomes mandatory for planners, practitioners, and laypersons to be cognizant of potential hazards as well as benefits. There is a potential for "lay professionalization." Policy studies should be encouraged on questions of the potential range of abuses; likely sources of abuse; and the requisite political, social, and administrative designs to serve as safeguards. What strategies can the health care establishment contribute to such policy development without destroying the essential core of self-care: its integrity as a lay movement.

International Strategies and the Avoidance of Chaos

The Copenhagen Symposium presented an interesting (and predictable) example of the many barriers to clear communication on the subject of self-care. Beyond the vagaries of the concept itself and differences in disciplinary perspectives, the cultural filter was the most obvious impediment as well as challenge to communication. Efforts to reduce the effect of this factor included joint planning sessions, background papers supplied in advance, specific work group agendas, work group summary reports, and plenary discussions. Certainly these devices were useful in ordering points for attention, but the very nature of self-care as a culture-bound phenomenon revealed the need for a more universal basis for discourse. Social and political perspectives as they reflected cultural differences also were evident sources of contention, producing shifts in levels of meaning of intent, often without warning. It was this obvious difficulty which stimulated consideration of the need for an international thesaurus, a classification scheme, or an information system as a prelude to developing reliable cross-national and cross-cultural research on self-care. At the very outset a central clearing house on self-care was seen as a way of producing a picture of the "state of play."

In effect, the Symposium group counseled that there is now a unique opportunity to avoid chaotic, parochial, and redundant research on a relatively new subject of international health interest.

The research ideas in self-care as reviewed here are offered in the context of an international undertaking involving, where feasible, cross-cultural comparisons. With the above requirements for a common "self-care language" in mind, there is every reason to expect productive joint enterprises among "lay groups" and scholars of many cultures. Indeed, the cultural variable itself may prove the most compelling and stimulating aspect of self-care development—how it determines self-care activity, how it directs change and filters choices, and how it influences the role of professional resources in health.

Who Should Be Involved in Self-Care Research?

Two points of controversy arose in the course of discussion on research challenges in self-care: the efficacy and role of "simple, cheap" research by health practitioners and others having continuous and direct access to lay populations; and the role of the layperson in the setting of objectives, design, conduct, and analysis of self-care research.

A proposal was made that the cumulative effect of self-care research would benefit by encouraging a broad range of studies to be undertaken at modest levels of financial and time investment. Here the group had in mind, for example, the opportunities for primary care practitioners to make limited but careful observations of patients—sometimes with the special advantage of close personal knowledge of the patients over a number of years. The point was made that self-care behavior as a field of study cannot rest solely on large population research which is particularly useful in describing normative behavior as differentiated by class, sex, age, and other demographic attributes. Clinical observations could provide a sensitive resource to test validity and to generate insights into the process and sequelae of self-care behavior. It is not a question of either-or, but rather to achieve a research undertaking which is balanced and opportune. Discussion on this point probably was merely a symptom of a larger underlying issue, i.e., establishing research boundaries or jurisdictions between clinician and social scientist. It was nonetheless useful in clarifying the need for a research policy on self-care which recognized that the nature of self-care behavior demands observation at several levels. At this point, a major burden of such a policy must be to stimulate research at the ground level, the level of direct client involvement. Case analyses, critical incident technique, participant observation, and other methods can make their contribution, by broadening the observation base and the range of research techniques applied.

Perhaps the most intense discussion of self-care research was focused on the role of the layperson. Several views were put forward which formed a rationale for lay involvement in self-care research. Central to this rationale is the concept of self-care as behavior which lies essentially outside the purview of the professional care system. As such, self-care relevant behaviors have not been defined, codified, or had efficacy levels determined. The demand for modifications or additions to self-care practices are not necessarily predictable on the basis of professional judgment of needs or appropriateness. Criteria of use, effectiveness, and demand may not, in effect, conform to the usual professional calibrations. It is necessary, therefore, to pursue a research strategy that will facilitate lay contributions to self-care theory-building (including rationale and benefits), and the identification of variables affecting self-care practices, the framing of hypotheses regarding self-care, and the setting of outcomes criteria.

Current health planning models typically do not account for the self-care factor; indeed the perspective is one of laypersons as "target" groups, passive recipients of service or as subjects for behavior modification efforts. Self-care research undertaken within the context of the current planning ethos appears more likely to test self-care practices as they fit the goals and needs of the professional care system than to test methods for adapting the professional care system to the self-care resource. These central concerns were expressed by several members of the Copenhagen Symposium, especially general physicians, who argued for a strong lay-professional partnership in self-care research through all phases of its design, execution, application, and evaluation.

Contrary views were put forward, not so much in opposition to the values expressed in the above position, but from the point of view that we should not fall into the trap of oversimplifying the complexities of research and the corollary requirements for research competence in a zeal to democratize the health care process. No one should be persuaded that research on self-care will require any less rigorous design and implementation than research on other aspects of social behavior. Indeed, it was emphasized that self-care research will be dealing with a wide range of unknowns, "soft" observations, and findings which will be subject to misinterpretation or misapplication unless their limits are tightly defined. This will demand rigorous and disciplined research regardless of who does it. But in the end, a participant noted, ". . . that research which reveals information that people find upon subsequent testing is correct is the research that will stand up."

References

[1] In order to determine the care provided as self-care, or for that matter the primary care provided by health professionals, a new descriptive terminology ("diagnosis system") is needed. The World Health Organization diagnosis list (International Classification of Diseases) is insufficient in describing some forms of morbidity, including social disability. What is needed is a system designed so as to be useful both for epidemiological analysis and as a basis for social planning and administrative practice.

[2] Lawrence L. Weed, *Medical Records, Medical Education and Patient Care* (Cleveland, Ohio: The Press of Case Western Reserve University, 1969).

[3] Lawrence L. Weed, *Your Health Care and How to Manage It* (Essex Junction, Vermont: Essex Publishing Co., 1975).

[4] John E. Ware, Jr., and Mary K. Snyder, "Dimension of Patient Attitudes Regarding Doctors and Medical Care Services," *Medical Care* 13 (August 1975), pp. 669–682.

[5] Thomas Szasz and M.H. Hollander, "A Contribution to the Philosophy of Medicine: The Basic Models of the Doctor-Patient Relationship," *Archives of Internal Medicine* 97 (May 1956), pp. 585–592.

[6] L.A. Aday and R. Eichorn, *The Utilization of Health Services; Indices and Correlates: A Research Bibliography* (Washington, D.C.: National Center for Health Services Research and Development, U.S. Department of Health, Education, and Welfare, DHEW Publication No. (HSM) 73–3,0003), 1972).

[7] Lois Pratt, *Family Structure and Effective Health Behavior: The Energized Family* (Boston: Houghton Mifflin Company, 1976).

[8] See "Self-Care in Health" Annotated Bibliography.

[9] Group-oriented self-care education programs could maintain continuous contact with clients over a period of time sufficient to evaluate the exigencies of self-care in practice; not only what was learned, but what proved useful in real situations. It would also be of interest to observe the ripple effect of self-care education as it is passed on to others in the family or community.

[10] See reference to Mary Ann Lewis' work at the University of California, Los Angeles, in the "Self-Care in Health" Annotated Bibliography, section on Risk Avoidance and Decision-Making.

[11] George G. Reader and Mary E.W. Goss (eds.), *Comprehensive Medical Care and Teaching* (Ithaca, New York: Cornell University Press, 1967).

[12] Herbert Menzel and Elihu Katz, "Social Relations and Innovation in the Medical Profession: The Epidemiology of a New Drug," in E. Gartley Jaco, *Patients, Physicians and Illness* (Glencoe, Illinois: The Free Press, 1958), pp. 517–528.

[13] Herbert F. Lionberger, *Adoption of New Ideas and Practices* (Ames, Iowa: The Iowa State University Press, 1960).

[14] One possibility in this regard is the development of new technology and industry around the production of materials and equipment purpose-built for self-care use. There is also the prospect of re-equipping home environments, e.g., adapting the bathroom to accommodate self-care functions.

[15] Lawrence W. Green, "Toward Cost-Benefit Evaluation of Health Education: Some Concepts, Methods, and Examples," Health Education Monographs 2 (Supplement), 1974, pp. 34–64.

Epilogue

It is said that the best ideas are those undergoing change. By such a test, this book must score high marks. Since we began the process of writing, and certainly since the Copenhagen Symposium in August 1975, the concept of self-care has blossomed in the public consciousness and belatedly, but inevitably, in academia as well. We have been stimulated (sometimes bombarded) with popular and scholarly works on the subject, and an amazing outcropping of self-care programs in the United States have come to our attention. Unfortunately, this volume had to close in the midst of what appears to be a rising tide (if not yet tidal wave) of interest and action in self-care.

As we look back at the Symposium and our elaboration and extension of ideas stimulated there, it is obvious that catching a social phenomenon in motion is a hazardous task. There were and still are few landmarks to give perspective in time; few precedents to calibrate the maturity of position; and hardly any secure language to communicate definite meaning. The intent of the Symposium and of this book was to begin to assemble ideas, conceptual tools, and strategies that give some measure of what is going on and might be anticipated. It is this latter aim which we tried to nudge a bit through various agendas of issues and prospects for research. We were confined largely to opinion and belief, buttressed by modest fragments of systematic observation and personal experiences. Accepted within these limits, this work may be useful to laymen, social scientists, and health professionals in stimulating imaginative inquiries and educational programs in self-care.

There surely will arise (and as of this writing we have heard some) statements of misgiving and concern about self-care and its promotion. Some health professionals sense an attack on their territorial rights while others are troubled by potential excesses in "going too far." An even more severe criticism is the possibility that self-care will be used as a pacification tactic to reduce public demand for more or better personal health services. In contrast, there are those who feel self-care is a middle class idea with little transferability to the interests of the poor. Others view self-care as a fad or a "reaction against" or as a protest that will pass from the scene once the cause(s) is won. And perhaps the most portentous concern comes from laypersons themselves: self-care may be co-opted by the health establishment.

Understandably there are and will continue to be diverse perspectives on and prognostications for self-care. Its ubiquity and persistence through history and its continuing vitality in controversy as well as practice are sufficient reasons for its study, but are they sufficient reasons for encouraging demonstration and further development? We believe the answer is "yes," with the caveat appropriate to all social interventions: *primum non nocere.* There clearly can be no guarantee of purity of intent, or benefits without deficits. But in the public interest the public must prevail, and as a popularly rooted phenomenon self-care's diversity and status as a civil right certainly will contribute substantially to maintaining its own integrity. This by no means suggests that we should be indifferent to the risks of self-care to clients, professionals, and laypersons generally. On the contrary, those concerns may be integral to the concept and may constitute at least an aspect of the social ecology of self-care and the interrelatedness of effects one might anticipate in its development. There are issues of balance society must calculate in assuming benefits over risks, not only in strictly "health terms" but also in relation to economic investments and displacement.

Aside from the many reasons put forward for the current focused interest in self-care, the realities of its necessity can be expressed in terms of its basic or essential functions to promote the public health, control preventable disease, manage chronic illness, and reduce iatrogenesis. Even within such minimal requirements for individual health care competence one is forced to consider public access to concepts and skills now partially or wholly within the control of health professionals. Through necessity more than public demand, many of these skills have been maintained by or transferred to the lay domain, but many—perhaps the most crucial ones—yet remain contingent on professional ministration. The morality of this situation, much less its rationality, is in serious question. Here there can be consensus on the default of the health care establishment to vigorously pursue the transfer of essential health care skills to lay responsibility. The irony is that many health professionals have only marginal interest in providing such technical services or are unable logistically (time and distribution limitations) to do so.

The trend of morbidity and the trend of medical practice appear to be coalescing with concurrent (1) public interest in reducing costs and iatrogenesis (clinical and social); and (2) advances in medical technology which make them more amenable to lay use.

This amalgam of circumstances, far from a conspiracy, is the product of social change, not its cause.

What appears to be occurring is a growing recognition of the holism of health and health care; a perspective which broadens the definition of health services resources to include that vast proportion of care laypersons now provide to themselves. At the same time the concept of health service itself has changed from a narrowly defined notion of the delivery of health skills to one which includes a variety of social, political, and environmental skills as well. In effect, all of this has contributed to a profusion of resources and, concomitantly, a diffusion of options. The core attribute of self-care is the process of posing the relevant questions (consciousness of interests and needs) and deciding what options are available and most promising of yield with the least likelihood of undesirable side-effects. Under such circumstances an erosion of resource monopolies in health activity is inevitable with a resulting loss in various areas of professional control. Further, predictability of the lay response to specific categories of the professional health resource will be increasingly difficult to achieve. Both health practice and health planning modules will need to respond to widening degrees of freedom in lay decision-making and evaluating service (including self-service) choices. Thus the study of self-care must be considered not only in the circumspect terms of an individual's behavior, but as the study of a broad and far-reaching revision in society's definition and use of its helping institutions. Self-care in health may be merely the first manifestation of this revision where parallels in education and social welfare can be expected to emerge in days immediately ahead.

Finally, we would like to reiterate the central point of self-care as a reality and as a resource of great promise. Its contribution to health care is not only supplementary to and substitutionary of currently available health care resources—it is *additive* to society's ability to overcome many extant barriers to health care accessibility, acceptability, quality, and accountability. In this sense self-care must be viewed as the *first* option, with any alternative being supportive and residual. It has always been so. The difference now is we are able to conceptualize the self-care option with more clarity than in the past. We have a new opportunity to consider how to further strengthen the lay contribution and at the same time make more precise and responsible use of technical-professional expertise in health.

"Self-Care in Health" Annotated Bibliography

Development of a bibliography on self-care was begun in preparation for the Copenhagen Symposium on The Role of the Individual in Primary Health Care. Participants in the Symposium contributed additional references as the concept of self-care was considered in increasingly broader terms and issues. On several occasions participants stated the priority importance of organizing information on self-care and designing an international system for sharing data. This annotated bibliography is an initial effort to assemble such references and is intended as a jumping-off point in the literature for scholars and practitioners of self-care.

The references selected for annotation from over 350 undertaken may represent only a small fraction of the relevant literature on self-care if one takes into account the wide range of concepts and technologies involved in health practice, many of which are integral aspects of culture, socialization, and survival. Indeed, it may well be that the most significant contributions to self-care thinking and practice could be drawn from anthropology, history, and philosophy and, of course, the popular literature of our times. In this sense, any effort to construct a bibliography on self-care is subject to the bias of one's own construction of reality. The additional problem of approaching a new and loosely defined field for inquiry and development causes a good deal of uncertainty with regard to coverage and representation. Such conditions tend to press the reviewer toward reliance on a literature which, on the whole, proclaims itself to be germane to self-care practice. The listing here must, therefore, be offered as a modest beginning more suggestive than definitive. Criteria for selection were our notion of relevance, originality, potential for research ideas, applicability to self-care program development, or contribution to conceptual growth. One or several criteria might apply in each case.

There were specific areas of coverage which received little or no attention because of their availability elsewhere (consumerism in health policy and systems operation) or because their extensivity or pervasiveness demanded a complexity of sampling and analysis beyond the resources available to us (self-care in the popular press).

Finally, we must note the very marginal inclusion of non-

United States literature. Anticipated companion efforts at the University of Nottingham Department of Community Health and University of Copenhagen-U.C.L.A. Joint Center for Studies of Health Programs at the University of Copenhagen will provide valuable supplementation to the present annotations.

Annotations are arranged under headings where judged most appropriate, but it is clear that there is often overlap in content across several categories. Hopefully, the annotations are sufficient to at least hint at these possibilities.

This bibliography was selected from the joint productivity of the authors and twenty-five graduate students at the Yale University School of Medicine, Department of Epidemiology and Public Health, during the period of January 1975 through May 1976. The authors are most grateful to the following students of self-care for their enthusiasm and persistence in a literature search which often required extraordinary ferreting skills: Joyce Adler, Jerry Ainsworth, Carol Battin, Pamela Berger, Barbara Bloom, Carolee DeVito, Deborah Dwork, Joyce Glazer, Patricia Golden, Beth Goldman, Karen Gordon, Bruce Grogan, Ellen Jaslow, Teri Klein, Lois Kwitman, Vivian Leslie, Sheldon Levy, Beverly Morrow, Alonzo Plough, Wayne Rems, James Roistacher, Steven Schwartz, Robert Silten, Barbara Unterman, and Barbara Wessen.

Concepts Central to Self-Care

Benham, Lee, and Benham, Alexandra. "The Impact of Incremental Medical Services on Health Status, 1963–1970." *Equity in Health Services: Empirical Analyses in Social Policy.* Edited by Ronald Andersen, Joanna Kravits, and Odin Anderson. Cambridge, Massachusetts: Ballinger, 1975, pp. 217–228.

This study tests the assumption that increasing medical services will result in improved health of the U.S. population. Using data taken from comparable national surveys conducted by the Center for Health Administration Studies, 1963–1970, they found incremental benefit to be small or negative even though in a specific instance benefits may be large. The authors point out that increased expenditures by the government on medical services can be counterproductive in that they draw resources away from more effective programs. Levels of education were found to be related to better health status. The authors conclude that such results should shift the burden of evidence to those who support increases in medical services as a means to improve the health of the general population.

Carlson, Rick J. *The End of Medicine.* New York: John Wiley and Sons, 1975, 290 pp.

Carlson reviews the assumptions of scientific medicine and develops a critique concerning the effectiveness of the medical care it provides. In the light of evolutionary analysis, the medical care system is viewed as being divergent from an emergent zeitgeist—a major societal transformation. A holistic medicine, calibrated with this new paradigm, is outlined that can replace the old model, which may self-destruct as a result of its own internal contradictions.

Foucault, Michel. *The Birth of the Clinic: An Archaeology of Medical Perception.* New York: Vantage Books, 1975, 215 pp.

Foucault presents a broadly based historical inquiry into the evolution of a particular medical paradigm, clinical knowledge. The formalization of clinical experience is seen as a reorganization of the spontaneous practice of health care by individuals and a variety of lay practitioners. The clinic represents a structural experience with an emphasis on "illness" as defined by an emerging medical elite. The role of this new model in the social control functions of the state is clearly explicated.

Freidson, Eliot. *Profession of Medicine.* New York: Dodd, Mead, and Co., 1973, 409 pp.

This is a classical work on the profession of medicine. Chapters on the professional construction of illness, the lay construction of illness, the limits of professional knowledge, and the limits of professional autonomy are central to the conceptual development of self-care. It is a clear and persuasive analysis of the social control of medicine and its consequences for the profession and the society which has provided its sovereignty.

Fuchs, Victor. *Who Shall Live?* New York: Basic Books, 1974, 168 pp.

Economist Victor Fuchs examines the American medical system, points out shortcomings, and presents recommendations for their solution. The author studies the relationship between health—as measured against a variety of socioeconomic indicators, e.g., education, income, life-style, etc.—and medical care. Components of the medical care system examined in detail are: physicians, hospitals, and drugs. Recommendations presented are designed to have a significant impact in the areas of cost and access. Topics covered are: health insurance, decentralization of delivery system, capitation payments, competition, use of allied health manpower, and hospital use. The author points out, however, that the implementation of these recommendations will do little in producing a significant change in the overall health of the population. This work clearly shows that life-style and general health habits have a greater influence on the general health of Americans; more so than increasing expenditures in medical services. The implications in the fields of health education and self-care are made obvious as the author concludes "the greatest potential for improving health lies in what we do and don't do for and to ourselves."

Illich, Ivan. *Medical Nemesis: The Expropriation of Health.* New York: Pantheon Books, 1976, 294 pp.

In this American edition of the previously published British version, Illich critically examines the medical institution and its structural insults to human health. Medicine is viewed as a metaphor which reflects the systemic counterproductivity that permeates the institutions of industrial production. In this system, "health" is reduced to a commodity. The resultant expropriation of mutual care and human coping ability creates an iatrogenic medicine that represents a pernicious force with clinical, social, and cultural ramifications.

Pratt, Lois. *Family Structure and Effective Health Behavior: The Energized Family.* Boston: Houghton Mifflin Company, 1976, 230 pp.

A provocative, perhaps survivalist attempt at reinvigorating family health behavior through an exploration of health and health behavior as a part of family sociology that proposes the theoretic construct of the energised family. If the family can still be considered a primary locus of socialization, then the importance of structural interrelations that can inculcate personal activation and provide a self-care milieu obtains. Essentially the thesis emerges that the traditional stable American family system serves to sustain medicine as an agent of social control. Families are seen as preparing all members for active confrontation with community agencies—butting a personal confidence against the formal technical system.

Pratt, Lois. "The Significance of the Family in Medication." *Journal of Comparative Family Studies* II (Spring 1973), pp. 13–31.

This paper reviews the literature in an attempt to correlate social factors with control over medication in a family. Areas covered include the extent of illness in families, the extent of medication, and the social forces controlling medication behavior. The author concludes that, at least in the United States and Great Britain, "professionals" control most health care functions. Families do, however, carry on a great deal of medicating which represents a power struggle between them and the health care bureaucracy.

Zola, Irving K. "Pathways to the Doctor—From Person to Patient." *Social Science and Medicine* 7 (1973), pp. 677–689.

This paper discusses the paths to becoming a patient following the perception of illness and taking into account any delay in deciding to seek help. Zola conducted a study of three ethnic groups at Massachusetts General Hospital (Boston) to determine their symptomatic perception of illness from listening to their complaints. The chief concern of this study was examining how the decision was made to seek help.

Historical Perspective

Alcott, William A. *The Home-Book of Life and Health; or The Law and Means of Physical Health.* Boston: Phillips, Sampson and Co., 1856, 500 pp.

This book, by an enormously popular physician, is a singularly complete work on the rules and laws of health and hygiene in everyday life. It encompasses a discussion of current mortality and morbidity rates in the United States, the state of commonplace health practices, and organ systems and their related diseases. The anatomy and physiology of the respiratory, digestive, and circulatory systems are explained to provide the base upon which he builds his theory of the healthy life. Emphasis is on the effect of everyday habits on the body. Occupational hazards, the problems of ventilation, methods of preventing consumptions, cookery and food, clothing, exercise, and rest are all of interest to the author. The book is clearly written and easily understood, but its main virtue is the simplicity with which it presents the 19th century model life style.

Alcott, William A. *The Young Housekeeper or Thoughts on Food and Cookery.* Boston: George W. Light, 1839, 424 pp.

The purpose of this book is to improve physical condition through nutrition. To do this, Dr. Alcott believes it is necessary to elevate the important profession of those for whom the book is written. Women, in their role as housekeepers, have many important functions; they are teacher, educator, counsellor, minister, etc. This treatise, however, deals mainly with the importance of basic principles of nutrition and cookery. A great variety of foodstuffs are discussed at length. The proper methods of preparation are described and the relation between the article of food and its effect on health is discussed.

This is an exhaustive discussion of 19th century principles of nutrition.

Alcott, William A. *The Young Mother or Management of Children in Regard to Health.* New York: James C. Derby, 1855, 342 pp.

This book on the proper care of the healthy child includes a discussion of appropriate and inappropriate food and drink, but there is also considerable attention given to the physical nature of the nursery, ventilation and control of temperature, the child's dress, the necessity of cleanliness and bathing, exercise, and rest. Nor is the author interested solely in physical welfare of the child. The physical state of the child is seen as necessary for his or her emotional well-being.

This book is clearly written and the information is presented in an orderly, logical fashion. To the 20th century reader its charm lies in the clear delineation of model 19th century child care principles and practices, and, consequently, in the resultant child model.

Beecher, Catherine E., and Stowe, Harriet Beecher. *Principles of Domestic Science.* New York: J.B. Ford and Co., 1870, 390 pp.

This book is written "for the use of young ladies in schools, seminaries, and colleges." Its purpose is to raise the level of education with regard to domestic science, its aim to improve the life of the Christian family.

This is a practical book. Floor plans, ventilation plans, furniture designs, and anatomy illustrations are carefully drawn to scale. The relationship between hygiene, housing, mode of life, and physical and mental health is stressed.

At the time of its publication this was an extremely important and comprehensive "how-to" book. Much of what is said is applicable today.

Chavasse, P.H. *The Physical Training of Children.* Philadelphia: New World Publishing Co., 1871, 368 pp.

This book, written in Platonic dialogue style by an English physician, deals with the proper care of the child from infancy, through childhood, and including boyhood and girlhood. This is a volume of advice and instruction written for the intelligent, but as yet ignorant, mother. A great deal of attention is given to clothing, diet, toilet, exercise, and sleep during the phases of childhood. Common ailments and diseases during each phase are also discussed, with special attention given to the recognition and diagnosis of symptoms. Considerable attention is devoted to the prescriptions and administration of medicines, and minute directions given for the arrangement and management of the sick room.

Fonssagrives, J.B. *The Mother's Work With Sick Children.* Translated from the French by F.P. Foster, M.D., Fourth Paris Edition. New York: G.P. Putnam's Sons, Handy Book Series, *ca.* 1872, 242 pp.

This book is from the Putnam's Handy Book Series. It deals in the main with cautions against practices injurious to health: charlatans, belief in gossip, useless and dangerous medicines. The author attacks popular misconceptions about phlegm, wind, worms, and humors and explains how these theories were developed, but does not explain why they were discarded. Dr. Fonssagrives devotes some time to explaining the hazards of dentition and growth, prescribing certain articles to be maintained as a domestic pharmacy in a locked medicine chest. He lists the symptoms of common pediatric ailments, but does not propose any treatment. Finally, he exhorts women on what observations to make regarding their children's growth and health stature, how to arrange a sick room (particularly the bed), what to wear while nursing, how to arrange administration of medicine and baths, the application of poultices and blisters, and suitable diet for a sick child.

This book illustrates what was then considered a baseline knowledge, and it is surprising to the 20th century audience to note that a woman who could not learn to use a thermometer was yet expected to make medicines according to exact formulae, and to know a great deal about herb baths, teas, and poultices.

Jacobi, Abraham. *Infant Diet.* New York: G.P. Putnam's Sons, Handy Book Series, 1891, 119 pp.

This treatise was first delivered by Dr. A. Jacobi before the Public Health Association of New York on May 8, 1873. It was subsequently revised, enlarged, and adapted to popular use by Mary Putnam Jacobi, M.D. This edition, written for a lay audience, is more than a dictum on the proper infant diet, explaining the physiological and chemical principles upon which theories of diet are based. Dr. Jacobi challenges common beliefs, explaining how they had come to be regarded as true and why they were false. He then proposes an alternative theory giving logical, easily understood reasons. For example, Dr. Jacobi explains that although mothers' milk is usually the best possible infant food, it must be understood that human milk is not a divine substance but a chemical composition which may or may not be appropriate.

Parker, Edward H. *The Handbook for Mothers: A Guide in the Care of Young Children.* New York: Hurd and Houghton Co., 1866, 250 pp.

This "safe and sufficient guide" to the management of children views the mother's role as limited primarily to preventive intervention, and that of the physician, to acute care.

Beginning with the care of the foetus and ending with the child in his or her sixth year, diet (nursing practices, wet-nurses, and artificial feeding, both substance and method), toilet, dress, education, and exercise of both mother and child are of major importance. Equal attention is given to recognizing symptoms of disease, with particular emphasis on different types of constipation, diarrhea, and coughs. Remedies for each illness and symptom, as well as remedies for emergencies such as earaches, dentition, burns, sprains, etc., are given. The course of action and medication is clearly described, including such minor surgery as lancing the gums of a teething child.

Uffelmann, Jules. *Manual of the Domestic Hygiene of the Child.* New York: G.P. Putnam's Sons, 1891, 228 pp.

This book, translated from the German by Harriet Milinowski and edited by Mary Putnam Jacobi, M.D., is "for the use of students, physicians, sanitary officials, teachers, and mothers." The original treatise was addressed to "Students, Physicians, Sanitary Officials, and Pedagogues," but the translator and editor address it to intelligent non-professional women as well.

This book is unusual in that it devotes to girlhood and boyhood the same careful attention it gives to infancy and early childhood. Anthropometry and normal physical standards are of great concern to the author as are methods of nourishing; there are detailed discussions of various cereals and other manufactured foods including statistics regarding results of their use. Dr. Uffelmann also devotes a great deal of attention to the care of the skin, respiratory organs, osseous and muscular systems, and the nervous system. Furthermore, he considers the questions of the hygiene of housing and intellectual and mental health.

This is a thoughtful, well-written, and detailed study of various aspects of childhood. Although it deals more with primary care of the child than with disease and remedies it puts a great deal of useful knowledge at the reader's disposal and presents in a logical fashion what was previously considered "too scientific" for the lay woman, and consequently obscured by commonplaces, vapid generalizations, and ignorance.

Cultural Differences in Self-Care

Currier, Richard L. "The Hot-Cold Syndrome and Symbolic Balance in Mexican and Spanish-American Folk Medicine." *The Cross-Cultural Approach to Health Behavior.* Edited by L. Riddick Lynch. Rutherford, New Jersey: Fairleigh Dickinson University Press, 1969, pp. 255–274.

An exposition of the Hot-Cold Syndrome and how it is used to explain the etiology of various diseases by members of Latin cultures. Folk treatments for these diseases also are discussed.

Saunders, Lyle, and Hewes, Gordon. "Folk Medicine and Medical Practice." *The Cross-Cultural Approach to Health Behavior.* Edited by L. Riddick Lynch. Rutherford, New Jersey: Fairleigh Dickinson University Press, 1969, pp. 402–408.

This paper discusses the extensiveness of the folk medicine network which, the authors maintain, constitutes a well-organized and consistent theory of medicine. These beliefs are not supplanted by scientific beliefs; rather, scientific beliefs are adjusted and fitted into the folk medicine structure. The authors point to the importance of the medical establishment's recognition of this fact and their consideration of folk medicine in treatment.

Lay-Professional Relationship (Personal)

Belsky, Marvin S., and Gross, Leonard. *How to Choose and Use Your Doctor.* New York: Arbor House, 1975, 240 pp.

This book is subtitled "Beyond the Medical Mystique, The Smart Patient's Way to a Longer Healthier Life." It is a good attempt at de-mystifying the physician. Geared to the literate middle classes, the book is full of real-life examples of do's and don'ts in physician-patient contact.

Freese, Arthur S. *Managing Your Doctor.* New York: Stein and Day, 1975, 191 pp.

The reader is admonished to be in control of his/her own health care. Everything is covered from choosing the doctor to special problems of females, elderly, and homosexuals. The physician is the technician and the consumer is the patient who needs to know how to manage the technician. The usual "bad medical machine" issues are ignored, and appropriately so, as the goal is to increase the communication abilities of the consumer. There is a useful medical library appendix of "books that will help you manage your doctor."

Gaver, Jessyca. *How to Help Your Doctor Help You.* New York: Pinnacle Books, 1975, 344 pp.

An excellent book for preventive episodic and chronic illness self-care. Information is provided to help individuals write and carry their own health histories, select a physician, determine the quality of the health care received, select modes of financing health care, and organize and maintain personal health records.

Griffenhagen, George B. "For a Better Informed Patient." *Journal of the American Pharmaceutical Association* 14 (December 1974), p. 665.

The article endorses the position of a committee composed of members of the American Society of Internal Medicine and the American Pharmaceutical Association Academy of General Practice of Pharmacy. This group is making formal policy decisions to urge pharmacists to work with local prescriber groups in an effort to implement broad guidelines. The ultimate goal of the enhanced communication is a "better-informed patient." Guidelines refer only to increasing the amount of information to be included on prescription order forms (and hence increase the directions and warnings typed on prescription labels).

Griffith, H.W. *Instructions for Patients.* Philadelphia: W.B. Saunders Company, 1975, 360 pp.

"This collection of instruction sheets presents a simple method of putting into the patient's hands pertinent material about his medical problem." The notebook is designed for the purpose of enabling a physician to give an instruction sheet on a particular illness or condition to the patient. The instructions are in lay language with brief explanation of the illness and why a medication is being used to treat it. Diets for special conditions, e.g., pregnancy, are also included as are simple diagrams of areas of the body, e.g., throat. A good index provides a quick reference.

Levin, Arthur. *Talk Back to Your Doctor.* Garden City, New York: Doubleday and Company, Inc., 1975, 245 pp.

The subtitle of this book is "How to demand (and recognize) high quality health care." The advice seems largely directed at middle class America and as such reflects the level of ignorance and mystification surrounding health care shared by laypersons of all walks of life. The author emphasizes the crucial role of the informed consumer in judging health care quality, choosing a doctor, understanding the diagnostic and treatment procedures, and in general gaining more control over the health care process. Rationales and implications of the process are summarized in "principles" that direct the reader to a specific action-conclusion or point relevant to the patient's decision-making.

Pratt, Lois; Seligman, Arthur; and Reader, George. "Physicians' View on the Level of Medical Information Among Patients." *American Journal of Public Health* 47 (October 1957), pp. 1277–1283.

The problems of communication between patients and doctors are examined to determine how effectively the doctor communicates with patients on important factors relating to illness, etiology, treatment, and prognosis. It was found that the level of understanding of these major elements was very low. In no single case did satisfactory knowledge of these areas exist. The authors note that there is a latent desire on the part of patients to have more knowledge of their illness and a desire on the part of doctors for their patients to receive such information. Improved communication is seen as a *sine qua non* for improving patient care.

Consumer-Provider Relationship (Administrative)

Cron, Theodore O. "A Patients' Revolt: Is it Possible?" *Hospital Progress* 51 (October 1970), pp. 69–71.

As president of the American Patients Association, the writer presents the purposes of the organization and lists the reasons for seeking change outside the health and medical professions. A Health Bill of Rights is presented at the conclusion of the article.

Friedman, J.W. *A Guide for the Evaluation of Dental Care*. Bethesda, Maryland: National Institutes of Health, Division of Dental Health, 1972, 93 pp.

The book describes the basic content of dental care and provides a method of direct and indirect evaluation of dental care quality. It was designed for use by dentists, administrators, and the public. The consumer is considered an integral part of the process, as is the dentist. However, the patient role is also felt to require change to a more active and informed one.

Gartner, Alan. "Consumers as Deliverers of Service." *Social Work* 16 (October 1971), pp. 28–32.

This article discusses both positive and negative practices employed by human service agencies to meet increasing demands for services. The author feels that the potential effectiveness of using the service consumer as a service deliverer should be included as a positive strategy for change. He cites several examples of self-care that have used this strategy.

Gartner, Alan, and Riessman, Frank. "The Consumer: A Hidden Resource for Improving Health Service." *Urban Health* 3 (December 1974), pp. 13–14, 46–47.

This paper presents a coherent argument for the idea that better health care can only be accomplished by consumers becoming operative in the delivery of the service. Several examples of self-care are cited.

Reeder, Leo G. "The Patient-Client as a Consumer: Some Observations on the Changing Professional-Client Relationship." *Journal of Health and Social Behavior* 13 (December 1972), pp. 406–412.

This paper is concerned with the changing professional-client relationship as a result of the development of consumerism in American society. The issue of consumer representation on various levels of the provider services also is discussed. Consumer participation is viewed as having two functions in health: planning and organization. Although the paper deals primarily with these issues in relation to health, it is seen as being applicable to other social issues.

Stacey, Margaret. "Consumer Complaints Procedures in the British National Health Service." *Social Science and Medicine* 8 (August 1973), pp. 429–435.

The author examines the problems inherent in the National Health Service for the development of complaint procedures, identifying obstacles that need to be overcome such as: the lower status of patients and their inability to complain effectively, fear of reprisals, the hierarchical structure of the health care system, the insistence of certain groups on clinical autonomy in decision-making, and lack of expression of effective consumer viewpoint at decision-making levels. Suggestions are offered for improving the responsiveness of the system to consumer demands.

Risk Avoidance and Decision-Making

Hansen, Fleming. *Consumer Choice Behavior.* New York: The Free Press, 1972, 548 pp.

The background on consumer behavior and decision-making provides a theoretical orientation for individual choice in decision-making patterns. Although the book is more oriented to consumers and "market" behavior, the implications and application for health behavior (as presented from several models of behavior) can be extracted. An extensive bibliography on choice behavior is provided.

Lewis, Mary Ann. "Child-Initiated Care." *American Journal of Nursing* 74 (April 1974), pp. 652–655.

In this study a nurse practitioner "describes an experimental system in an elementary school which encourages children to decide on their own when they need to seek care and to participate in decisions on managing their problems." Although the author states that the anecdotal evidence from the study suggests that this type of decision process has had the desired effects, no statistical information is presented.

Mayer, Jean. *Health.* New York: D. Van Nostrand Company, 1974, 532 pp.

This book was designed as the text for an introductory college course in health. It contains articles by the author's colleagues at Harvard, each writing in his or her area of expertise. Subjects fall into the categories of human biology, medicine and preventive medicine, public health, and human ecology. The material is presented with photographs, illustrations, and interesting margin notes. This book provides a broad framework of understanding health in a social and ecological context.

Mead, Johnson and Co. *A Safe Home for Your Children.* Indiana: Mead, Johnson and Co., 1967.

This pamphlet provides parents with a basic knowledge of potential environmental dangers. Briefs concerning accidents and their relationship to the various age groups are presented to guide the parent with regard to high risk factors. Preventive aspects are emphasized and the caretaker is given full responsibility for the enactment and maintenance.

Pinckney, E.R. *You Can Prevent Illness.* Philadelphia: Lippincott, 1960.

A comprehensive guide for health care, protection, prevention, and maintenance of the family. The expected topics are covered—occupational health, immunizations, periodic exams—but also there is, unusually, coverage of eye health and environmental factors. Each chapter ends with a list of specific recommendations for personal action. Emphasis is given to the primary responsibility of the individual in disease prevention and the need to change habits, seek information, and demand service. Professional health care providers are placed in the perspective of a secondary (to the individual) care resource.

Roth, Julius. "Who's Complaining." *Trans-Action* (July/August 1965), pp. 12–16.

Need for a health complaint mechanism for improving the responsiveness and accountability of our social institutions has led the author to undertake an extensive examination of present system reactions to complaints. Methods to develop more skillful complainants within the citizenry and to improve abilities in effectively registering complaints are discussed and priorities of need and changes in the system are suggested.

Sobel, David. *Everyday Guide to Your Health.* New York: Grossman Publishers, 1973, 190 pp.

Directed toward a lay audience, the *Everyday Guide to Your Health* is intended as a resource to be used to educate individuals to care for themselves. The emphasis is toward the maintenance and improvement of health, rather than the treatment of specific ailments. Presented as a series of exercises, the reader is provided with information regarding health practices directly related to life-style, e.g., eating habits, breathing, relaxation, body movement, etc. Not intended as a substitute for medical intervention, the basic premise is that through adoption of the health practices presented, the need for medical intervention will be greatly diminished.

Spencer, David, and Lloyd, John. *A Child's Eyeview of Small Heath Birmingham: Perception Studies for Environmental Education.* Birmingham, England: Centre for Urban and Regional Studies, University of Birmingham, 1974, 171 pp. (Research Memorandum 34.)

The short descriptions of Small Heath based on school children's observations and comments provides insight into what are outstanding environmental problems of the area. The use of a "sensory walk" through a neighborhood or street suggests an educational approach to developing skills of critical evaluation of an individual's immediate environment. The Bibliography on Environmental Education is very comprehensive.

Stellman, Jeanne, and Baum, Susan. *Work is Dangerous to Your Health.* New York: Vintage Books Division, Random House, 1973, 448 pp.

This handbook, written for the layman, covers information about a variety of work environments, what elements are generally present and what effect they have on the individual's health, and what the individual can do about them. The book gives suggestions on how the individual or group, e.g., of miners or factory workers, can do something about occupational hazards.

Whelan, Elizabeth M. *A Baby? Maybe: A Guide to Making the Most Fateful Decision of Your Life.* New York: Bobbs-Merrill Co., Inc., 1975, 237 pp.

This is a discussion of parenthood and pregnancy, intended as a consciousness raiser in the need for planning and budgeting for children. Practical information is given to insure intelligent planning, such as a balance sheet to impel qualitative decision-making and the ability to justify whatever decision is finally made. Of interest to self-care because of the application of decision theory.

Women's Yellow Pages: The Original Source Book for Women. Boston: Boston Women's Collective, Inc., 1973, 159 pp.

A yearly referral source book for and to various people and agencies mainly in the Boston area, but is of more general interest as a prototype approach. The health care section in addition to the usual gynecological emphasis provides information about homemaker and visiting nurse services, sickle cell disease, and mental health. There is an interesting section on aging that might have been developed further.

Self-Observation

Frank, Arthur, and Frank, Sutton. *The People's Handbook of Medical Care.* New York: American Book—Stratford Press, 1972, 494 pp.

The goal of this book is to help laypersons assume responsibility for their own care as well as to inject a social perspective into their discussion of medical problems.

Hansen, M.F., and Reib, K.G. "An Educational Program for Primary Care: An Outline of a Curriculum." *Journal of Medical Education* 45 (December 1970), pp. 1007–1015.

Though this paper does not deal directly with self-care or patient education, its potential applicability to both should be considered. An outline for the training of primary practitioners is presented. Concepts of the patient and his body in relation to disease are well organized within the outline. The epidemiological approach seems to have been a strong influence. Less detailed and technical versions of this outline could become the basis for patient self-care education courses.

Mellner, Christian. "The Self-Administered Medical History." *Acta Chirurgia Scandinavica,* Supplementum 406, Malmö, 1970, 104 pp.

Dr. Mellner examines some of the theoretical possibilities and practical limitations of the usefulness of a self-administered medical history. An experiment to test this approach was undertaken at the Malmö General Hospital in 1967–1969, to examine the type and frequency of technical errors, reliability of information obtained, and variation in physicians' evaluation. Although the subject of self-care is not directly considered, the implications of this system can be translated in this context. The journal is helpful for examining such issues as the role of the patient in planning a medical examination if a significant amount of the work can be performed by the patient himself.

Rodale, Jerome I. *Encyclopedia for Healthful Living.* Emmaus, Pennsylvania: Rodale Books, Inc., 1960, 1,056 pp.

The author provides a potpourri of preventive and self-care techniques from the naturalist's perspective. Cures and/or preventive suggestions are given for over 3,000 diseases or infirmities ranging from abortion to hemorrhoids. The basic assumption is that all illness can be prevented and/or cured with special diet, frame of mind, or exercises prescribed in the book.

Shenkin, Budd N., and Warner, David C. "Giving the Patient His Medical Record: A Proposal to Improve the System." *New England Journal of Medicine* 289 (September 27, 1973), pp. 688–692.

The authors develop a proposal to give the patient his medical record as a device to improve patient information, increase consumer opportunity to exercise free choice in selecting physicians, increase patient autonomy in decision-making, improve quality of care through improved accountability, and increase patient satisfaction. The problems of fragmentation, specialization, increased centralization and control, and potential improvements of the system are discussed.

Sorochan, Walter D. *Personal Health Appraisal.* New York: John Wiley and Sons, Inc., 1976, 302 pp.

This book is designed for college students with a focus on assessing and modifying personal health. It includes a variety of scales and inventories for self-analysis that cover the total health spectrum. There is a section on biochemical tests and behavior modification modules that address personal physical and mental health.

U.S. Department of Health, Education, and Welfare. *Breast Self-Examination.* Washington, D.C.: Government Printing Office, 1972.

The writers of this pamphlet present a pictorial step-by-step protocol for breast self-examination. However, the layperson's role is described exclusively as one of detection, leaving the individual in a passive-receptive role through the treatment and management phases.

U.S. Department of Health, Education, and Welfare. *Cancer Questions.* Washington, D.C.: Government Printing Office, 1966.

This pamphlet presents a brief synopsis of risk factors and the various cancers. The purpose, effectively achieved, was to provide the reader with a more accurate data base and dispel some of the myths of cancers.

Weed, Lawrence. *Your Health Care and How to Manage It.* Essex Junction, Vermont: Essex Publishing Co., 1975, 194 pp.

A "do-it-yourself" guide to record evaluation by the originator of the problem-oriented medical record. The book contains useful information on the components of the medical record and guidelines for evaluating it. A cooperative patient-physician relationship is assumed, and sample records are provided as illustrations. The "Health History Questionnaire" included as an appendix could serve as an excellent guide for patients who want to keep their own records.

Self-Diagnosis

Bates, Barbara. *A Guide to Physical Examination.* Philadelphia: J.B. Lippincott Co., 1974, 375 pp.

This is a standard textbook of physical diagnosis used by nurse-practitioners. It provides complete basic information on physical examination with numerous illustrations of anatomy and examination techniques. Two drawbacks are lack of information about using diagnostic equipment and no explanations of the significance of abnormal findings. If supplemented by a good medical text, this would be an appropriate guide for the home physical examination.

Gomez, Joan. *A Dictionary of Symptoms.* New York: Stein and Day Publishers, 1972, 398 pp.

A complete outline of common physical symptoms for the layman. This is a quick desk reference for the home. Its treatment sections tend to be scanty, however. There is a basic assumption of responsibility on the reader's part to evaluate symptoms and encourage understanding of the processes that produce symptoms.

Mariken, G. *A Doctor's Sensible Approach to Alcohol and Alcoholism.* Chicago: Bud Long Press, 1969, 97 pp.

The terms and vocabulary are for readers at and above the middle class level. An historical development is presented on the abuse of alcohol. The physiological effects are well detailed. A sufficient data base is acquired, so that the reader may determine if he or others are having drinking problems.

Neubardt, Selig. "How to Examine Your Breasts." *Cosmopolitan* (May 1975), p. 90 passim.

A discussion of the importance of breast self-examination, and a thorough step-by-step procedure for the woman to follow.

Skydell, Barbara, and Crowder, Ann. *Diagnostic Procedures: A Reference for Health Practitioners and A Guide for Patient Counseling.* Boston: Little Brown and Co., 1975, 248 pp.

A short book written in outline form with many photographs and diagrams of equipment and procedures. Common diagnostic tests such as mammograms are briefly explained in terms of purpose, preparation, equipment, and patient sensations. This is a clearly written reference for the patient who wants to be fully prepared for diagnostic procedures.

Yankaur, Alfred; Johnson, Anita; Stim, Edward M.; and Ibrahim, Michael A. "Do-It-Yourself Pregnancy Testing." *American Journal of Public Health* 66 (February 1976), pp. 129–133.

Four articles are presented explaining the legal and medical positions on Ova II. The papers are short, precise, and helpful to the person anxious to know the status of Ova II as an acceptable self-administered pregnancy test.

Self-Treatment (General)

American Red Cross. *American Red Cross Home Nursing Textbook.* 7th ed. New York: Doubleday and Co., Inc., 1974, 368 pp.

The first edition of this handbook was published in 1913. Except for its acknowledgment of more recent scientific advances especially in the area of rehabilitation and disaster care its useful presentation has probably changed little since it was first published. The book is meant to accompany Red Cross classes on home care and does a good job of helping "home nurses" recognize illnesses and handle a plethora of nursing procedures.

Beland, I., and Passos, J. *Clinical Nursing.* New York: Macmillan, 1975, 1,099 pp.

An approach to clinical nursing which is based on a systems approach to patient care. A wide variety of health disorders are discussed on the basis of physiological systems such as "The Patient with a Problem of Nutrition." Using concise explanations of pertinent anatomy and physiology as a base, the authors discuss each problem in terms of prevention, diagnosis, and treatment. All problems are considered within the context of the "whole person" with psychological and environmental factors well defined. Although hospital-oriented, this is an excellent reference text for layperson and health provider alike.

Bennett, Hal Z., ed. *The Well Body Student Health Manual.* Berkeley, California: University of California, 1974.

This booklet gives general "tips" relevant to "common health problems." Topics are geared to campus health and sickness situations: minor diseases, sex and contraception, preventive living (learning to relax, eating well).

Boston Women's Health Book Collective. *Our Bodies, Ourselves: A Book By and For Women.* 2nd ed., revised and expanded. New York: Simon and Schuster, 1975, 383 pp.

This enormously useful and valuable book has been revised and expanded since its first printing in 1973. Even with additions and changes, the authors emphasize that much of the information will soon be outdated. However, the carefully compiled resource lists which follow each section make it an easy task to follow up on specific information or to seek additional information about any topic(s).

Sections which have undergone complete revision are: Sexuality, Common Medical and Health Problems, Venereal

Disease, Rape, Abortion, Considering Parenthood, Preparation for Childbirth, Some Problems in Childbearing, Menopause, and Women and Health Care. The changes reflect the growth in the writers, the suggestions of readers, and the many changes in the health field itself.

This collaborative effort on the part of many women to learn about their own bodies and share their knowledge with other women is clearly written, offering excellent technical information on anatomy and physiology (and explanations of how the scientific terms equate with popular usage or slang expressions) as well as supplying the reader with short anecdotes from the lives, thoughts, and emotions of many women. This work goes far beyond an indictment of the medical profession as it delineates areas of neglect or misunderstanding of women's bodies and feelings on the part of professionals. While it points to the problems (e.g., the potential harmful effects of estrogen replacement therapy for menopausal women, or the incidence of vaginal cancer in the adolescent daughters of women who were given DES to prevent spontaneous abortion), it also explains which kinds of problems are amenable to professional treatment, many problems and procedures that can be handled by women themselves, what kinds of treatment women should seek, how to select the professional source of treatment, and how to be an informed patient who will be herself a part of the treatment program. Thus the book is also an invaluable source for the *professionals* who are concerned with women as patients.

In the final chapter, "Women and Health Care," questions of women's health needs are related to the larger question of the American health care system.

Browder, S. "What to do About Those Ubiquitous Vaginal Infections." *Cosmopolitan* (February 1976), p. 106 passim.

All the common causes of vaginal infections are covered. The presentation is easily read and understandable. The causes, symptoms, and treatment types, side effects and benefits are well developed. The section of what to do and not to do, leaves the individual in control and allows for a partner-relationship with the health care provider.

Cooper, Kenneth. *Aerobics.* New York: M. Evans and Co., Inc., 1968, 253 pp.

This book suggests the development of endurance and fitness by increasing oxygen consumption, strengthening heart and lung activity. According to the author, the best exercises are in this order: running, swimming, cycling, walking, stationary running, handball, basketball, and squash. Large team sports are not as good, but better than calisthenics and weight lifting. Program adopted by the United States Air Force. May be somewhat strenuous for the average person.

Copans, Stu, and Osgood, David., eds. *The Home Health Handbook.* 2nd ed. Burlington, Vermont: La Pauvre Press, 1971, 200 pp.

This manual provides, in lay language, information relevant to health and sickness situations and is specifically directed to rural residents and commune communities. Precise information, often with diagrams, is offered with respect to preventing, recognizing, and treating health and illness situations. Subjects covered range from first-aid to venereal disease to stress, drugs, safe canning, and home delivery of babies.

Corrigan, A.B. *Living with Arthritis.* New York: Grosset and Dunlap, 1971, 146 pp.

The aim of the book is to help the patient and family understand various common skeletal diseases and the appropriate treatment, so that the individuals can better adapt and become informed consumers. Non-medical therapies are viewed as quackery and the reader is warned of the dangers of these alternatives to medical therapy. The language is easy to understand, illustrated with patient cases, but lacks the necessary diagrams for a complete understanding.

D'Alonzo, C.A. *Handbook of Heart Disease, Blood Pressure, and Strokes.* New York: Collier Books, 1960, 127 pp.

Opposing views are presented as the author warns the reader against self-diagnosis and ignorance of the causes, treatment, and prevention of cardiovascular diseases. The book was written for the consumer. It provides a good data base for the individual to understand the significance of symptoms, when to seek care, and, once in the realm of medicine, what and why things are being done.

Dolger, H., and Seeman, B. *How to Live with Diabetes.* New York: Pyramid Books, 1965, 192 pp.

An excellent reference for the patient and his family. All aspects, including the psychological and how to buy medications cheaply, are covered in detail. The book can help develop a more educated and activated individual.

Gemini Collective. *The Gemini House Manual: A Comprehensive Primer on Drug and Life Information.* Chicago: Salsedo Press, 1975, 159 pp.

A complete and professional manual by a storefront drug clinic collective in Champaign, Illinois. It deals with physical and emotional drug interactions and dependence. The emphasis is on the street drug trade with specific precautions and instructions for emergencies but it is of interest to anyone who would help someone in trouble. Nutrition, patients' rights, birth control, V.D., and abortion as well as an extensive local referral list are all dealt with appropriately and provide real tools for those interested in self-help in these areas.

Gould, Heywood. "How to Soothe an Aching Head." *Woman's Day* (March 1976), p. 32 passim.

Massaging is presented as a safe, simple, and quick way to relieve headaches. The massage as medication is not always the only solution but this alternative form is less expensive and dangerous to your health.

Harvey, A. McGhee, et al., eds. *The Principles and Practices of Medicine.* 18th ed. New York: Appleton-Century Crofts, 1972, 1,650 pp.

A clinical approach to diagnosis and treatment used by professional readers as a supplement to Harrison's *Principles of Internal Medicine.* Diseases are discussed in symptomatic groups such as "Upper Respiratory Infections." Emphasis is on a step-by-step diagnostic approach and management techniques. Simple explanations of physiology with diagrams are included. Although knowledge of medical terminology is required, this is probably the most useful standard medical reference for the layman.

Ishmael, W.K., and Shorbe, H.B. *Care of the Back.* Philadelphia: J.B. Lippincott Co., 1955.

This pamphlet presents excellent illustrations and explanations of medical jargon and therapies. The focus is for the self-care aspects of back care. There are lists of do's and don'ts for daily prevention and treatment of existing problems. The recommendations are practical and easily incorporated into a daily routine.

Jarvis, D.C. *Folk Medicine: A Vermont Doctor's Guide to Good Health.* New York: Henry Holt and Company, 1958, 182 pp.

This book represents an exploration into Vermont folk medicine practices. As such, it provides an insight into the self-care interventions which are commonly practiced by a large group of rural residents. Jarvis explores the efficacy of these treatments and how they should be used when specific symptoms are in evidence.

Migraine Information for Patients. New Jersey: Organon Press (Number R944).

The differences between the migraine syndrome and symptoms is outlined. What is a migraine is clearly described and its variability is stressed. The types of attack are sketchily presented. Enough information is given to whet an appetite, but not enough to understand the dynamics involved. Anatomy is dispersed throughout the pamphlet, but without adequate visual aides. The triggers of attacks are listed, so that the individual can try to identify the precipitating factors of one's own migraine. Treatment and prognosis are mentioned without any detail. The recommendation to keep a diary of episodes is useful to aid the individual in management of attacks.

Orem, Dorothea. *Nursing: Concepts of Practice.* New York: McGraw-Hill, 1971, 237 pp.

This book is a well-articulated theoretical explanation of self-care and its relationship to the nursing profession. Self-care is presented as the optimal baseline for the population. Self-care activities are defined in terms of characteristics, decision-making, and action. Nursing is defined as an art which assists people when they cannot care for themselves and gradually returns them to self-care status through support and teaching. A complex but well-reasoned conceptualization of the components of self-care and their relationship to one of the health professions.

Paulsen, Kathryn, and Kuhn, Ryan A., eds. *Woman's Almanac: 12 How-To Handbooks in One.* Philadelphia: J.B. Lippincott Co., 1976, 624 pp.

This book is a storehouse of valuable and useful information on many topics, including physical and emotional health, sexuality, education, work, business, money management, legal problems, politics, and simple home repairs, among others. Sections dealing with health advice, first aid, childbirth, abortion, contraception, gynecological surgery, menstrual problems and menopause, immunizations, drugs and medications, adoptions, together with discussions of depression, anxiety, self-analysis, consciousness-raising groups, assertiveness training, creative dreaming, comprise almost half the book. A "Woman's Directory," called the "Woman's Yellow Pages," at the back of the book lists over 1,500 local and national women's services and organizations. Some of the articles were written for this book; others are reprinted from a wide variety of sources.

A section specifically labeled "self-care" is disappointingly small—a brief comment by a woman physician on the use of the speculum by self-help women's groups. However, much of the information can be applied toward the care of one's self, can help the individual to make wise choices when professional sources of care are necessary, and can direct the reader to additional sources of information.

Romney, Seymour, et al. *Gynecology and Obstetrics: The Health Care of Women.* New York: McGraw-Hill, 1975, 1,163 pp.

A revolutionary textbook which portrays women as human beings rather than just pelvic organs. The whole range of obstetrical and gynecological problems are discussed lucidly as a symptomatic approach with good illustrations. Excellent chapters on psychosocial problems such as "Bioethical Debates in Gynecology and Obstetrics" are included.

Rosenthal, Richard. *The Hearing Loss Handbook.* New York: St. Martin's Press, 1975, 222 pp.

The purpose of creating awareness of improvement, as contrasted to procedures used by "professionals" which may increase the sense of the handicap of hearing loss. The ultimate goal is to promote the controlling patient, not the controlled.

Practical advice predominates throughout, producing an excellent source book for persons with hearing losses and their families.

Royal Canadian Air Force Exercise Plans for Physical Fitness. (U.S. ed.) New York: Simon and Schuster, 1962, 80 pp.

Short illustrated pamphlet. Variations on five basic exercises for men and ten basic for women. Requires 11–12 minutes a day. Program simple. Self-reassuring. Person progresses at his or her own pace through series of levels. As with any home plan, motivation is a large factor.

Rush, Anne Kent. *Getting Clear (Body Work for Women).* Berkeley: Random House Bookworks, 1973, 290 pp.

"Body awareness" through exercise and discussion is the thrust of this book on female energy. The book's emphasis is on reclaiming one's body from others and learning alternate ways of handling stress and pain.

Samuels, Mike, and Bennett, Hal. *The Well Body Book.* New York: Random House, 1974, 349 pp.

Written for the layman, this book is an excellent resource for any self-care curriculum developer. Content includes: taking a medical history, health implications of daily living habits, and common minor illness recognition and treatment. In the minor illness section, each topic is discussed, when appropriate, as to (1) observable signs and symptoms; (2) other symptoms to look for; (3) what's happening in the body when one feels ill; (4) treatment measures the individual can take; and (5) the doctor as a resource.

Schmidt, Alice M. *The Homemaker's Guide to Home Nursing.* Provo, Utah: Brigham Young University Press, 1976, 181 pp.

A mixture of custodial nursing and first aid written in the nurse-patient idiom. The author prefaces the book with her observation of the inadequacies women of all ages feel toward dealing with illness in the home and thus provides a domestic nursing primer for the "home nurse," referring to any family member who is giving the nursing care. The book covers home nursing skills, first aid, the process of aging, lifting and caring for the bedridden, convalescent care of sick children, facing terminal illness with family members, and disaster preparation.

Sehnert, Keith W., with Eisenberg, Howard. *How to Be Your Own Doctor (Sometimes).* New York: Grosset and Dunlap, 1975, 353 pp.

This is probably the most comprehensive and well organized—and practical—guide to medical self-help available. A rationale for self-help (the "activated patient") sets the stage for the guide to lay intervention in common illnesses, common injuries, most common emergencies, a drug index, treatment index, symptom/concept index, and testing index. A listing is included of self-help brochures, guides, pamphlets, and other materials useful in building self-help concepts, knowledge, and skills.

Spock, Benjamin. *Baby and Child Care.* Newly Revised, Updated and Enlarged. New York: Pocket Books, Inc., 1968, 620 pp.

Dr. Spock has again revised his classic manual to mold to the changing times, reworking especially his attitudes toward male/female roles. He provides a comprehensive discussion of the special problems of infancy, the normal child at various ages, parenting advice on behavior, nutrition, and routine care. Less emphasis is given to sick children. The author carefully advises "consult your doctor"—even at very safe stages in the progression of children's illness. He insists: "Don't give medicine without a doctor's advice and don't continue it without keeping in touch with that doctor . . . Parents who have treated colds or headaches or stomach aches a few times in the same way come to feel like experts, which they are in a limited way. But they're not trained, as a doctor is to first consider carefully what the diagnosis is."

Stolten, Jane. *Home Care: A Guide to Family Nursing.* Boston: Little, Brown and Company, 1975, 400 pp.

This book addresses itself specifically to the nursing care of the ill or feeble person at home. It offers some good suggestions on the safety, exercise, bathing, and diets of bedridden patients. The appendix includes a definition of types of physician (dermatologist, etc.) and a list of national organizations that can be used as resources for more information on nursing care of the home bound.

Thosteson, G. *The Everyday Medical Handbook.* Greenwich, Connecticut: Fawcett Publications, Inc., 1974, 70 pp.

The author presents an accumulation of commonly asked medical questions from his newspaper column. The physician is seen as the key to diagnosis and management, with the consumer as a passive recipient. In terms of the health content, the responses are accurate, useful, and dispel many myths.

Vickory, Donald M., and Fries, James F. *Take Care of Yourself.* Reading, Massachusetts: Addison-Wesley Publishing Co., Inc., 1976, 269 pp.

The subtitle of this manual is "A Consumer's Guide to Medical Care." Using an algorithm approach, the authors concentrate on nearly seventy health problems both commonly seen and often commonly misunderstood. Background on each health procedure or health problem is cogently presented in lucid, jargon-free terms and includes statements concerning the limits of our knowledge—having the salubrious effect of demystifying and humanizing the issue involved. The book is arranged in sections: Skills for the Medical Consumer, The Patient and the Common Complaint, and Family Records. Locating the appropriate subject is as simple as determining your chief complaint or symptom. Of special usefulness are ample discussions on how to manage the health care system, although advice regarding following doctors' instructions tends to take a simplistic view of the doctor-patient relationship, with a major cause of a poor relationship being identified as the recalcitrant patient.

Wilson, Judy. *Mother Nature's Homestead First Aid.* Willits, California: Oliver Press, 1975, 152 pp.

A cleverly illustrated and simply written first aid manual designed for a new breed of country dwellers—urban immigrants. The book, therefore, concentrates on emergencies which the urbanite may have taken to an emergency room but now, without such resources, must take care of on his own. Special attention also is given to risks associated with country living—snake and viper bites. Recommended emergency procedures reflect the practicalities of the rural environment and ordinarily available materials and tools.

Self-Medication

Ames, Richard. "How to Survive a Heart Attack." *Readers Digest* (November 1973), pp. 110–114.

A clearly presented discussion of heart attacks—why they occur, how to recognize the early warning signals, and what to do to give yourself the best chance for survival and recovery. The individual is presented with a complete plan of action once the "diagnosis" of his/her heart attack is made.

Burack, Richard. *The New Handbook of Prescription Drugs.* New York: Ballantine Books, 1975, 440 pp.

This book is an informative and handy guide through the maze of prescription drugs. There are lists of drugs with descriptions, commentaries, and cross-references; price lists with druggists' costs; and basic pediatric prescription drugs. Dr. Burack makes his case both for the use of generic drugs and for more thorough training in pharmacology for physicians. The message and facts are worthwhile and would be of use in self-care education programs.

Consumers Union. *The Medicine Show.* New York: Pantheon Books, 1974, 384 pp.

This is a useful reference for choosing drugs and drug products based on facts other than those from drug manufacturers. Over the counter (non-prescription) and prescription drugs are presented in relation to common problems such as colds, dandruff, and arthritis. "How to" chapters include choosing a hospital and doctor, and stocking a medicine chest.

DiCyan, Erwin, and Hessman, Lawrence. *Without Prescription.* New York: Simon and Schuster, 1972, 321 pp.

With respect to commonly acquired disease states, this book describes effective drug entities and their effects. It refers to chemical ingredients rather than referring primarily to specific trade name products. Thus, it allows the reader to extrapolate newly acquired knowledge to various products.

Feldmann, E.G. "OTCs: End the Dual Standard." *Journal of Pharmaceutical Sciences* 62 (April 1973), I.

The author calls on the pharmacy industry and profession to ensure efficacy and quality of over-the-counter products as well as offering as much advice and counseling to the OTC purchaser as the prescription purchaser. He points out that "the pharmacy profession . . . has found itself influenced by what might be termed the 'condescending attitude' that the medical profession assumes toward the self-medicating patient." He refers to the self-medicating patient as a reality and self-medication as a valid part of the health care system.

Fox, Lloyd A. "Written Reinforcement of Auxiliary Directions for Prescription Medications." *American Journal of Hospital Pharmacy* 26 (1969), pp. 334–341.

This article is essentially a listing of precautions and prescription drugs to which they are applicable, presenting very necessary and beneficial information to accompany products dispensed. Presentation of information is straightforward and lacks unnecessary sensationalism.

Griffenhagen, George B., and Hawkins, Linda L., eds. *Handbook of Non-Prescription Drugs.* American Pharmaceutical Association Publication (annually since 1967).

The editors make the generalization that "self-medication" is an integral part of health care today. Over-the-counter preparations are listed under general therapeutic categories. Product name, manufacturer, dosage form, and ingredients are listed for comparison along with a general narrative in each category. Material is provider-oriented with the assumption that this publication "will continue to better equip the pharmacist and other members of the health professions with facts to make the self-medicating public a little safer and non-prescription drugs a little more useful."

Stress Management

Beary, John, and Benson, Herbert. "A Simple Psychophysiologic Technique Which Elicits the Hypometabolic Changes of the

Relaxation Response." *Psychosomatic Medicine* 36 (March/April 1974), pp. 115–120.

During the practice of an easily learned relaxation technique, oxygen consumption, carbon dioxide production, and respiratory rate are significantly decreased. These changes are consistent with an integrated "tuning down" of the sympathetic nervous system—a suggested counterpart of the "fight-flight syndrome." Elements of the technique are outlined in the article: a mental device to prevent distracting thought, a passive attitude, decreased muscle tonus, and a quiet environment. Simple instructions for eliciting the relaxation response are presented.

Benson, Herbert. *The Relaxation Response.* New York: William Morrow and Co., 1975, 158 pp.

The book is concerned with the cause and effect relationship of stress on the human being and a simple meditative technique to relieve the symptoms of stress through mental relaxation. Physiological data are presented as a basis for recommended methods.

Hamburg, David; Coelho, George; and Adams, John. *Coping and Adaptation.* New York: Basic Books, 1974, 454 pp.

Edited collection of studies and views of means of coping with stress both from a biological and social perspective. Provides a broad theoretical framework for considering stress management as an active process over time.

Jacobson, Edmond. *You Must Relax.* New York: McGraw-Hill, 1962, 269 pp.

The author suggests that in the technique of progressive relaxation, the person seeks to achieve increased discriminative control over skeletal muscle until he is able to induce very low levels of tonus in muscle groups. Jacobson states that anxiety and muscular relaxation produce opposite physiologic states and therefore cannot exist together. The subject is taught to recognize even slight contractions of muscles so that he can avoid them and achieve a deep degree of relaxation. Somewhat long procedure to learn.

Newman, Mildred, and Berkowitz, Bernard. *How To Be Your Own Best Friend.* New York: Ballantine Books, 1971, 91 pp.

A "do-it-yourself" approach to personal mental health, written in dialogue form for the layman. The book avoids the usual discussion of mental illness, and in simple terms presents positive, although perhaps oversimplified, principles of skill development for mental health.

Raymond, Margaret; Slaby, Andrew; and Lieb, Julian. *The Healing Alliance.* New York: W.W. Norton and Co., Inc., 1976, 287 pp.

This book by a social worker and physicians (one a psychiatrist with public health background) is an interesting discussion on the use of families for psychiatric therapy when one of their members is disturbed. It covers the role of the family and various treatment approaches.

Selye, Hans. *The Stress of Life.* New York: McGraw-Hill Book Co., 1956, 324 pp.

Provides an understanding of stress as it affects our physical and emotional states. Defines stress as a syndrome consisting of all the non-specifically induced changes within a biologic system, essentially the rate of wear and tear in the body caused by life. Scientific explanation of general adaptation syndrome (GAP)—body response to stress. Suggested coping methods are theoretical. Presents "deviation theory": equalize stress by shifting work of body from one part to another. Suggests optimum speed of living varies for each individual.

Selye, Hans. *Stress Without Distress.* Philadelphia: J.B. Lippincott, 1975, 171 pp.

This book has 136 pages of text plus a glossary of scientific terms and an extensive bibliography. The author offers a concept of stress as an essential part of motivation and experience. An attempt is made to correlate the general adaptation syndrome and measurable cellular response to emotional and physical body response. The author presents a philosophy of altruistic egotism and the need and yearning to be productive to "earn thy neighbor's love."

Shepard, M. *Someone You Love is Dying.* New York: Harmony Books, 1975, 218 pp.

The discussion is of death and dying, but a large section of the book is devoted to the role of hospitals, nursing homes, and hospices. The alternatives to self-care in the home are explored.

Physicians are presented as ordinary people with fears and desires like anyone else. The role of the professional is to offer symptom relief, not control of the total individual. An easily understandable presentation of how to be one's own advocate is included with available resources.

Signell, Karen. "Parent-Child Communication Course." *Exchange* 1 (April 1973), pp. 50–53.

This article describes a primary prevention model for mental health. The purpose of the course is to transmit to parents communication skills they can use with their children in everyday situations at home. Some of the mothers who went through the course became group leaders for future courses. The concept of mutual self-help for parenting is proved effective. The effectiveness, however, is presented in an anecdotal manner with no supporting data.

Viscott, David. "Free Yourself from the Oppression of Bad Moods." *Today's Health* 52 (March 1974), pp. 24–27, 61–63.

The author gives advice on how to improve mental health by learning to understand feelings, and how to control moods through positive mental exercises. An oversimplified, but interesting do-it-yourself program for mental health.

Human Sexuality

Campbell, Elizabeth. *A Woman's Beginning Guide to Self Health and Sexuality.* Colorado Springs, Colorado: Circle One, P.O. Box 7211, 1975.

A short introductory booklet that deals with issues of sexuality and health. Topics of pelvic examination, vaginal infections, birth control, abortion, cancer, and childbirth receive superficial, yet sensitive treatment.

Heidenstam, David, ed. *Man's Body: An Owner's Manual.* New York: Paddington Press, Ltd., 1976, unpaginated.

This book uses a format similar to *Our Bodies, Ourselves* (Boston Women's Health Book Collective). It has multiple graphs, scientific illustrations, and information on contraception and sexual intercourse as well as a discussion of the effects of alcohol and exercise on one's body. Cardiovascular risks and disorders are the traditional health information areas covered.

Rorvik, David. *Good Housekeeping Woman's Medical Guide.* New York: Good Housekeeping Books, 1974, 309 pp.

Good information is presented about anatomy and sex (called sex and common sense). This is a factual yet pristine book about women's "most intimate concerns" written in the style of women's magazines. It provides good information that might appeal to an audience that would not be reached by more earthy discussions.

Self-Care for the Elderly

Chandler, Robert; Eslinger, Elizabeth; Mackler, Margaret and Selkin, James. "A Geriatric Treatment Philosophy." *Journal of the Fort Logan Mental Health Center* 3 (Winter 1965), pp. 79–86.

Article describes goals and program of Fort Logan's first geriatric unit, begun in October 1964. Basic approach is remotivation toward productive social relations with emphasis on self-help, mutual aid, self-esteem, and confidence regarding the future. Treatment includes social therapies, insight therapies, activity therapies, and medical therapies.

DiCicco, Lena, and Apple, Dorrian. "Health Needs and Opinions of Older Adults." *Sociological Studies of Health and Sickness.* Edited by Dorrian Apple. New York: McGraw-Hill Book Co., Inc., 1960, pp. 26–39.

This paper represents an inquiry into how older adults (over 65) perceive their personal health needs and their attitudes toward the health care delivery establishment. The authors found that the elderly held the conviction that aches, pains, and physical limitations are an integral part of old age and, consequently, were not likely to seek formal medical interventions. The paper also explores the differences between those elderly who do seek medical care and those who do not.

Smith, Elliott Dunlap. *Handbook of Aging.* New York: Barnes and Noble Books, 1972.

The author wrote this book for "those growing old and those concerned with them." Aging is presented as an age of problems whose solutions are often demeaning. However, there are presented certain solutions to problems the elderly may encounter; solutions which appear creative and require minimal adaptation to implement.

Walker, Morten. *Your Guide to Foot Health.* New York: Arco Publishing Co., 1974, 224 pp.

Safe home remedies for foot care are presented in the context of an informed and active consumer role. Preventive foot care is emphasized, where 85 percent of foot problems are self-inflicted and 95 percent are preventable. The description of foot anatomy and physiology is excellent. Various practical hints for prevention—buying shoes, foot exercises, and daily foot care—are included. Additionally, this book is appropriate for reference material when intervention of a physician is needed, so that the individual understands and can participate in the diagnosis and subsequent therapy.

Maternal and Child Care

Altshuler, Anne. *Books that Help Children Deal with a Hospital Experience.* Washington, D.C.: U.S. Department of Health, Education, and Welfare, DHEW Publication No. (HSA) 74–5402, 1974.

This pamphlet presents an annotated bibliography of books for children that discuss hospital experience and illnesses. In the introductory section, questions are posed in order to help parents, teachers, and health professionals decide whether the books meet the special needs of the individual child, present a realistic picture of the hospital experience, and are of good literary and artistic merit. The bibliography itself is excellent and points out both positive and negative aspects of each work.

Arms, Suzanne. *Immaculate Deception: A New Look at Childbirth in America.* Boston: Houghton Mifflin Co., 1975, 318 pp.

Although neither a medical textbook, a political treatise, or a birth manual, this book is the philosophical manifesto for "self-birth," natural childbirth which unlike many professional-oriented methods of prepared childbirth training (controlled distraction), allows a woman to participate in her body as it births itself, a deep and complete involvement of the female sensorium in the birth process. The American way of birth is described as stripping the birthing mother of control of her own birth with its technologized interventions, isolation, and ideal of painless, risk-free birth. The case is made for the option of natural homebirth where a midwife as protector of the normal and cautious critic of interference is solicited as the arm of simple patience and constant care.

Davis, F. "Who's Having the Baby—You or the Doctor?" *Woman's Day* (March 1976), p. 10 passim.

The article prepares the reader for the self-deterministic approach for childbirth. The description of the process, as now done, is detailed and well presented. Alternatives to this traditional approach are presented in detail.

Eloesser, Leo; Galt, Edith; and Hemingway, Isabel. *Pregnancy, Childbirth and the Newborn: A Manual for Rural Midwives.* Mexico: Instituto Indigenista Interamericano, 1955, 150 pp.

"A product of necessity" written as a basis of instruction for midwives (country women who could be taught simply and in a short period of time how to help and not harm women entrusted to their care) in remote parts of the developing world. Chapters on the anatomy and physiology of the female reproductive organs, step-by-step methodology on progress and conduct of pregnancy and childbirth, and care for the newborn, itemization of equipment and technique generously enhanced by diagrams, make this book an excellent manual for anyone who wants to know what happens and what is to be done during pregnancy. Despite its vintage, an important find for self-care.

Ewy, Donna, and Ewy, Rodger. *Preparation for Breastfeeding*. New York: Doubleday, 1975, 125 pp.

Realizing that breastfeeding is a skill of motherhood lost in a generation gap, the three keys to successful breastfeeding (knowledge, support, and preparation) are discussed. The preparation section includes diagrams and a photographic case progression showing the simple conditioning of the breasts in months prior to birth and then the step-by-step delineation of the nursing process. A synopsis focuses on frequent problems—signs, prevention, and practical suggestions—e.g., of poor supply, inhibited "letdown reflex," engorgement, sore nipples. Another appendix lists breastfeeding contacts for information and further suggested readings. Of all the books reviewed on breastfeeding, this is a singularly practical manual.

Ewy, Donna, and Ewy, Rodger. *Preparation for Childbirth.* New York: Signet, 1970, 224 pp.

A step-by-step diagrammatic exposition of the steps of delivery—the different contractions: effacement, dilatation, transition, expulsion, with the matching Lamaze relaxation and breathing exercises. The roles of both husband and wife are emphasized.

Feinbloom, Richard I. *Child Health Encyclopedia.* Boston: The Children's Hospital Medical Center, 1975, 561 pp.

This voluminous reference aims to strengthen the role of the parent as the key member of a comprehensive health care team, as provider of primary front line care for children against a well-knit backdrop of close, continuous medical support. The essay and safety sections provide a general informational grounding for parents in quality pediatric care; regular physical checkups; diets of infants and children; the emotional anxiety-transferring dimensions of complaints; caring for the sick child; the hospitalized child; and the broad picture of health care delivery. A section on first aid is organized for quick reference. There is an alphabetic glossary of childhood diseases and conditions to be used as the need for information arises. Specific symptomatic diseases are covered as well as larger social child health issues.

Gordon, Thomas. *P.E.T.—Parent Effectiveness Training.* New York: New American Library, 1970, 334 pp.

The tested, transactional method devised by a clinical psychologist to develop optimal parent-child relationships by means of constructive problem solving and active listening that mobilizes both the wisdom of the parent and the child and impels inner directed, self-initiated, responsible behavior in children. A philosophy of child rearing that de-mystifies parental authority and releases both parent and child for self-directed growth by replacing problem solution orientation with creative process methodology.

Hazell, Lester Dessez. *Commonsense Childbirth.* New York: G.P. Putnam's Sons, 1969, 243 pp.

A sensitive and comprehensive digest blending philosophy, experience, and step-by-step guidance for prospective parents with the art and science of natural, relaxed, family-centered childbirth. Antenatal care; how to choose a doctor and hospital responsive to the couple's views; preparations for homebirth; husband-coached birth; and childbirth exercises and breast-feeding techniques are discussed in full with appendices capsulizing frequent questions about birth, a quick reference labor guide, and emergency childbirth and community resources. A valuable manual in childbirth education.

Ingelman-Sundberg, Axel; Wirsen, Claes; and Nilsson, Lennart. *A Child is Born.* New York: Dell Publishing Co., 1974, 160 pp.

A discussion of the development of an infant from conception to delivery is excellent. Included in the pictorial essay is a description of the first and subsequent visits to the physician. The hows and whys of what takes place are clearly presented, although there is an occasional lapse into jargon.

Karmel, Marjorie. *Thank You, Dr. Lamaze.* New York: Dolphin Books, 1959, 195 pp.

The author presents a narrative of her experience with the Lamaze method of childbirth. The presentation of information is brief, clear, and accurate. The enclosed manual of information and exercises is not to be taken as an absolute but in conjunction with supervision of "trained" personnel. The role of the active parent is stressed.

Kitzinger, Sheila. *The Experience of Childbirth.* Harmondsworth, Middlesex, England: Penguin Books, 1972, 280 pp.

The book was written for the layperson as a new outlook on the normal process of pregnancy and childbirth. The theme is that pain and displeasure of childbirth and pregnancy are intimately related to fear and a lack of understanding of the process. Philosophy of shared parental joy is outlined in messages for expectant mothers and fathers. The physical process of birth is detailed with pictures, and the adjustment to a child is described.

Lang, Raven. *The Birth Book.* Palo Alto, California: Genesis Press, 1972, 158 pp.

The back-to-nature primer in homebirth, this self-care manual pictorially presents homebirth and itemizes equipment, books, herbal remedy and techniques of perineal massage and the delivery process, infant resuscitation, and, in its natural lot of enthusiasm, even includes a recipe for placenta stew. A total restitution of birth to nature and communal laity.

Levine, Milton, and Seligmann, Jean. *The Parents' Encyclopedia.* New York: Thomas Y. Crowell Co., 1973, 619 pp.

Many aspects of pediatric medicine are presented for the parent. In addition, there are interspersed adequate descriptions of the psychosocial changes through infancy and childhood. Instructions are clear and well illustrated. An excellent appendix of resource agencies in the United States is included.

Marzollo, Jean, ed. *Nine Months, One Day, One Year: A Guide to Pregnancy, Birth and Babycare Written by Parents.* New York: Harper Colophon Books, Harper and Row, 1975, 191 pp.

This parent-oriented manual is a reaction against books written by health professionals with *their* special biases. The only way to find any sort of peace and contentment in parenthood is, the editor contends, to find one's own way and do it "without guilt, without perfection, and without comparing oneself to others." Included is a pregnancy diary describing body changes in a journalistic case study; a listing of the available birth methods with the advantages and disadvantages of each; a glossary for routine checkups; birth case studies; mother care and baby care in the first year; welcoming rituals; a sickness and health section of short hints and recommendations; a discussion of problems in parenthood; a Bill of Rights for Parents; notes of mothers and fathers on child care responsibilities; infant paraphernalia advice; and, finally, an excellent annotated bibliography on books about pregnancy, birth, and baby care.

Pratt, Lois. "Child Rearing Methods and Children's Health Behavior." *Journal of Health and Social Behavior* 14 (March 1973), pp. 61–69.

This paper describes a study which explores the relationship between child-rearing models and personal health practices of children. A developmental pattern of child rearing was found to be better associated with health care practices by children than a disciplinary pattern of child rearing. The developmental methods included substantial use of reason and information, rewards, and granting autonomy. The health practices involved the child's resources and capacities for coping and taking care of himself.

Shiller, Jack G. *Childhood Illness: A Commonsense Approach.* New York: Stein and Day, 1972, 310 pp.

A warm, reliable and self-confidence building primer in do-it-yourself pediatrics, written by a pediatrician who wishes to topple the era of panic pediatrics and replace it with commonsense parental management of childhood illness. Decision thresholds are carefully articulated between self-managed, home-based treatment procedures and professionally required care based on lucid discussion of signs, symptomatology, and degree. A tincture of time and judicious neglect is often advocated to allow for composed self-resolution of illness before final retreat to the system. Chapters are action-oriented, arranged for easy reference.

Sidel, Ruth. *Women and Child Care in China.* Baltimore, Maryland: Penguin Books, Inc., 1972, 207 pp.

This is an overview of the recent Chinese revolution and its liberating effect on women. The process of liberation is presented from the perspective of improved health services, exceptional health education, and special attention to pre- and post-natal child care. The concepts of general health care are blended effectively with individual education, concern, and self-care. The main thrust of the book is the relationship of these practices to the political and social values underlying contemporary China.

Taylor, Grant. "Leukemia: A Guide to the Management of the Disease." New York: Leukemia Society of America, Inc., 1971.

This publication typifies pamphlets prepared in an effort to reduce parents' fears with respect to their child's condition. The pamphlet describes normal courses of therapy and procedures. Some resources on U.S. local and national levels are presented.

Tucker, Tarvey. *Prepared Childbirth.* New Canaan, Connecticut: Woman's Library, Toby Publishing, 1975, 143 pp.

A rather academic explanation and guide to labor/delivery, hospital procedures, training, techniques, medications, rooming-in, breastfeeding, choosing an OB—a guide for young couples who need to decide whether to pass through a "crisis or a peak experience." Of most interest is the preface by Virginia Beal, a noted childbirth educator, who describes her initial hesitation at endorsing such a book by a lay non-expert.

Ward, Charlotte, and Ward, Fred. *The Home Birth Book.* Washington, D.C.: New Perspective/Inscape Book, 1976, 149 pp.

An anthology of essays by "institutional" contributors describing the personal, medical, psychological, social, and practical dimensions of the homebirth experience. An attempt at social legitimation of homebirth by serious consideration of the question, is homebirth really safe? and the conclusion that, providing a mother is under a doctor's care and prognosis is for a birth with no complications, birth at home is actually safer for both mother and child.

Nutrition

Berkeley Women's Health Collective. *Feeding Ourselves.* Boston: New England Free Press, 1972. Order from Berkeley Women's Health Collective, 2214 Grove Street, Berkeley, California 94704.

This short, yet comprehensive work gives information on digestion, the basic nutrients, special diets, weight reduction, food for pregnant and nursing women, babies, how to conserve time and money, food preparation tips, and an annotated list of references. The pamphlet begins with a discussion of the American food industry including the Food and Drug Administration and ends with suggestions for consumer and political activities on food issues.

Goodhart, Robert S., and Shils, Maurice E., eds. *Modern Nutrition in Health and Disease: Dietotherapy*. 5th ed. Philadelphia: Lea and Febiger, 1973, 1153 pp.

Written as a reference guide for physicians and other professionals, this work contains invaluable information for those interested in applying the concept of self-care in the area of nutrition. The forty-one articles are organized into six sections: (1) The Foundations of Nutrition; (2) Safety and Adequacy of the Food Supply; (3) Interrelations of Nutrients and Metabolism; (4) Malnutrition; (5) Nutrition During "Physiologic" Stress; and (6) Nutrition in the Prevention and Treatment of Disease. The appendix includes diets for a number of diseases and conditions. There is an index. The work's technical language may make it less accessible to some readers.

Kirschmann, John D. *Nutrition Almanac*. New York: McGraw-Hill, 1973, 263 pp.

Written for a lay audience, *Nutrition Almanac* is designed to provide a comprehensive understanding of nutrition and its effects on health. The reader, through the use of various tables and charts, can design a diet based upon individual needs. Use of nutrients by the body is explained so as to afford the individual information necessary for an informed decision concerning his or her diet. Information given is explicitly described as being non-prescriptive. The reader is encouraged to seek professional assistance in cases of special diets or allergic reactions. Included is an extensive bibliography and a glossary of terms.

U.S. Departments of Agriculture and Health, Education, and Welfare. *Food Is More Than Just Something to Eat*. Washington, D.C.: U.S. Departments of Agriculture and Health, Education, and Welfare in cooperation with the Grocery Manufacturers of America, and the Advertising Council, unpaginated. Order from U.S. Department of Health, Education, and Welfare, Public Health Service, Food and Drug Administration, 5600 Fishers Lane, Rockville, Maryland 20852.

This excellent pamphlet is written clearly and very attractively illustrated. Besides providing basic information on the major nutrients and their sources, there are discussions of the nutritional requirements of various age groups including the pregnant woman, infants and children, adolescents, young adults, and older adults. There is an explanation of nutritional labeling, a daily food guide, and a discussion of the different social, geographical, and cultural traditions that influence American diets. A section on "The Value of Processed Foods" suggests the difference between this booklet and the previous work.

Winter, Ruth. *Beware of the Food You Eat.* New York: Crown Publishers, Inc., 1971, 247 pp.

The book is intended for lay readers and serves as a compendium of information about foods and food additives.

Dental Health

Ferris, R.T., and Winslow, E. "Reinforcing Desired Behavior with Peridontal Patients." *Dental Clinics of North America* 14 (April 1970), pp. 279–286.

The purpose of the article is how to strategically plan for patient education during treatment. The educational process presented for the patient is based on learning theory for what and when. Active patient participation was seen as an essential element for success. The authors provide an exemplary program and how to evaluate it.

Igbal, A. *Orthodontics—A Simple Doctrine.* Pakistan: Khyber Mail Press, 1971.

The book was written for dental students and takes a rather paternalistic view of the patient. Despite this, it is an effective general reference for any layperson contemplating dental treatment. Jargon and terms are well defined and the book is easily read.

Lantner, M., and Bender, G. *Understanding Dentistry.* Boston: Beacon Press, 1961, 214 pp.

The goal of presenting common dental facts for the public is accomplished by this volume. The illustrations are clear and vocabulary defined. The role of self-care is indirectly supported in the section on "Before You See Your Dentist." The book is an excellent reference text not only for prevention, diagnosis, and treatment but also on how to choose a dentist.

McBride, Walter C. "The First Twenty-five Years." *Journal of Dentistry for Children.* Fourth Quarter (1952), pp. 144–153.

An historical and humorous narration of dentistry today. However, it offers some helpful ideas to equip the layperson to participate more effectively in the management of dental care.

McGuire, Thomas. *The Tooth Trip: An Oral Experience.* New York: Random House, 1972, 233 pp.

This informative book, written by a dentist, takes much of the mystery out of dental care. Practical, simple measures for self-care of the teeth and mouth are emphasized, but also included are descriptions of professional care and means for evaluating dentists.

National Institutes of Health. *Canker Sores and Fever Blisters.* Washington, D.C.: National Institutes of Health Publication No. 72–247, 1972.

A well-presented article of etiology, symptoms, and treatment or lack thereof. Stress is on the role of the individual to self-treat through two weeks of active disease. The role of the physician or dentist at this point is clearly outlined.

National Institutes of Health. *Rx for Sound Teeth.* Washington, D.C.: National Institutes of Health Publication No. 76–793, 1976.

This pamphlet is a brief but succinct manual for preventive home dental care with good clear illustrations.

Revere, P. *Dentistry and Its Victims.* New York: St. Martin's Press, 1970, 305 pp.

A "devil's advocate" book written by an anonymous dentist for the layperson's enlightenment regarding organized dentistry. The second, and successful, purpose of the book is to provide the layperson with a handbook of dentistry and dental health.

U.S. Department of Health, Education, and Welfare. *Tooth Care.* Washington, D.C.: Department of Health, Education, and Welfare Publication No. (NIH) 74–449, Health, Education, and Welfare Consumer Information Series No. 1, 1974.

A rather simplistic presentation of dental care. The pamphlet describes the individual's role in prevention—how to clean your teeth, role of nutrition, and fluoridation. However, valuable information of what to do when a dental accident occurs is carefully and clearly detailed.

Wheatcroft, M.G., and Arnim, S.S. "An Effective Program of Oral Hygiene the Dentist Can Teach the Adolescent." *Dental Clinics of North America* 13 (April 1969), pp. 375–386.

A method to teach adolescents and other patients what they need to know to prevent and control caries and peridontal disease is presented.

Mutual Aid Groups

Bailey, Margaret B. "Alcoholics-Anonymous Groups as an Aid to Wives of Alcoholics." *Social Work* 10 (January 1965), pp. 68–74.

Describes Alcoholics-Anonymous as a fellowship for relatives and friends of alcoholics. Alcoholics-Anonymous theory starts with the idea that each alcoholic is likely to affect several family members, resulting in mutually destructive interaction. In the group, spouses and other family members can find aid in understanding the alcoholic, social support, new activities, new friends, and encouragement to scrutinize and change themselves.

Bales, R.F. "The Therapeutic Role of Alcoholics Anonymous as Seen by a Sociologist." *Quarterly Journal on Studies of Alcoholism* 5 (June-March 1944–45), pp. 267–278.

Alcoholics Anonymous described as a social organization analogous to a living organism. Organization serves as a reference group for the individual, providing common problems and experiences and a strong large-family solidarity centered around recruitment and maintaining soberness. Craving for a drink is combatted through underlying needs for adjustment, providing other means or activities, breaking up the obsession with drink, and acquiring more effective thoughts and feelings. Group breaks through individual's sense of isolation and distrust extending even to himself. Each response of the individual to the recruitment call is a basically religious act and binds him ever closer to the group.

Bumbalo, Judith. "The Self-Help Phenomenon." *American Journal of Nursing* 9 (September 1973), pp. 1588–1591.

A review of self-help groups that have succeeded as well as those which have failed. Criteria are given to evaluate the effectiveness of such groups, and a selected list of self-help groups is given.

Caplan, Gerald. *Support Systems and Community Mental Health.* New York: Behavioral Publications, 1974, 267 pp.

The author focuses on health-promoting forces which enable people to deal with the nature of stress, both its challenges and strains. The book describes the spontaneous social networks developed by informal neighborhood care-givers and the organized supports of mutual help groups and associations. It presents several models for the development of support systems within the community, drawing on the strength of already established informal social groups.

Cohen, F. "Alcoholics Anonymous Principles and the Treatment of Emotional Illness." *Mental Hygiene* 48 (October 1964), pp. 621–626.

The author discusses the applicability of the AA program to general psychiatric problems. AA's goals are trustful relation to a "higher power," willingness to confront painful past experiences, cooperation with peers, and aid to others. The program's technical features are the screening-out of unresponsive alcoholics, non-professional supervision, reciting of common experiences, group belongingness, and frequent meetings. Cohen sees positive results in stability of mood, sense of well-being, relief from anxiety and depression, and modified perceptions and expectations of others.

Dis-Coverer 2 (March 1965).

This issue of the *Dis-Coverer* is devoted to self-help organizations in the areas of alcoholism, drug addiction, and mental disturbance. Some groups briefly described are Hazelden, Minnesota; Daytop Lodge in New York; Recover, Inc. in Illinois; and Shadybrook House in Ohio.

Grimstad, Kirsten, and Rennie, Susan, eds. *The New Women's Survival Catalog.* New York: Berkeley Publishing Corp. for Coward, McCann and Geoghegan, Inc., 1973, 223 pp.

Using the format of *The Whole Earth Catalog,* this is a resource book for names and addresses of various feminist collectives, clinics, and other women's organizations. Included are annotated bibliographies and pictures. Its chapter on "self-health" lists the pertinent clinics, books, and pamphlets that seem to have proven effective as well as supportive to the women's movement across the United States.

Katz, Alfred H. "Self-Help in Rehabilitation: Some Theoretical Aspects." *Rehabilitation Literature* 28 (January 1967), pp. 10–30.

Discusses social phenomena underlying self-help movements, relates them to other current social trends, and examines use of self-help approaches in rehabilitative services. Author cites groups deprived of normal growth within mainstream of society who develop self-organization as alternative path to identity realization, constructive activity, and heightened social communication. He stresses the self-help group's capacity to counter bureaucratic "treatment" systems with social innovation, pioneering, and grass-roots expansion closely molded to the actual living situation, and predicts increasing use of self-help approaches.

Katz, Alfred H. "Self-Help Organizations and Volunteer Participation in Social Welfare." *Social Work* 15 (January 1970), pp. 51-60.

The article provides a theoretical analysis of the dynamics of self-help groups, e.g., those organizations initiated and led by persons having common problems, social needs, and purposes. It includes analysis of structural features, functional attributes, and the process of self-help group influence. An annotated bibliography entitled "Self-Help and Rehabilitation" reviewing social science literature relevant to self-help groups is available from the author.

Katz, Alfred H., and Bender, Eugene I. *The Strength In Us: Self-Help Groups in the Modern World.* New York: Franklin-Watts, 1976, 304 pp.

This work offers a wide-screen presentation of self-help groups both in the United States and other countries, combining case illustrations and theoretical analysis. The historical development of mutual aid or self-help activities, the current scope and forms of self-help organizations, their structural features, inner dynamics and meaning to members, their relationship with professionals, their probable future as alternative forms of service vehicles, are discussed by the authors and other contributors. While not focused on health groups specifically, the book deals with mutual aid groups' role in drug abuse and other addictions, and mental health issues.

Palmer, Mabel B., and Hoffman, E.L. "A Study of the Membership and Program of a Club of Ex-patients of Mental Hospitals." *Mental Hygiene* 48 (1964), pp. 372–379.

Authors interviewed some members of the Magnolia Club in New Orleans to investigate who benefits most from an ex-patient social club, which club program is best, and how members' relative success in the club can be judged. Characteristics of successful members generally were age 25–45; potentially employable; white collar, middle-class; at least high school education; short hospital term; and current psychiatric help. Success seems to be judged in terms of lack of rehospitalization and re-entry into the community. Goals within the club are growing self-confidence, friends, new social skills, and increased familiarity with the larger community.

Racker, Franziska W.; Delgai, E.F.; and Abramson, A.S. "The Therapeutic Community: An Approach to Medical Rehabilitation." *Archives of Physical Medicine and Rehabilitation* 44 (May 1963), pp. 257–261.

Two groups of physically disabled patients are compared in an experimental ward and a control ward using traditional rehabilitation procedures. Experimental ward stressed coordinated staff, round-the-clock program, group participation, patient self-determination and self-expression, participation of families in rehabilitation, community integration, and follow-up program. Traditional ward showed reduced initiative and motivation, fear of leaving hospital, inadequate interest in others, disruption of family and social ties, and post-hospital retrogression.

Rennie, Susan, and Grimstad, Kirsten, eds. *The New Woman's Survival Sourcebook.* New York: Alfred A. Knopf, 1975, 245 pp.

This book offers an extensive list of sources for women in such areas as health, work, education, literature, communications, the arts, religion, politics, and others. Each section includes well-written, informative articles as well as lists of agencies, books, publications, and services. Many of these are reviewed or annotated; and articles serve to relate the information to a larger area of concern.

A thirty-page section on health discusses the reclaiming of women's bodies by women, particularly women's self-help efforts to control their own reproductive processes. Among the topics presented are pregnancy and childbirth, birth control, abortion, breast cancer, drugs, nutrition, sexuality, and mental health. The articles are brief; the annotated lists of relevant books are current and inclusive. In all, this is a valuable resource for women in general, which includes useful information for women interested in self-care.

Schwartz, Marc. "Situation Transition Groups: A Conceptualization and Review." *American Journal of Ortho-Psychiatry* 45 (October 1975), pp. 744–755.

This paper reviews literature on common characteristics, modes of function, and problems of small discussion education groups. These situational groups are used in a variety of settings for the mutual assistance of individuals who share a stressful life situation. Although moderated by a leader who facilitates discussion, they are not therapy groups. Once started by a "leader," the group is then often able to continue on its own, drawing new leaders from the group. The author acknowledges that sound research on S.T. groups is scanty, but anecdotal reported results in the literature support their effectiveness.

The Source Collective. *Organizing for Health Care.* Source Catalog 3. Boston: Beacon Press, 1974, 249 pp.

This book is a compendium of methods, materials and groups which can ". . . assist the people challenging outmoded and oppressive institutions." As such, this sensitive and practical reference identifies a wide range of resources in health that meet health needs of clients while demanding minimum dependency or the sacrifice of integrity. A good number of the resource groups are self-help oriented. Similarly, materials (articles, films, tapes) are rich in information contributing to personal/ social growth, freedom, and protection. Categories of health resources also reflect the special needs of prisoners, the elderly, the deaf and hearing-impaired, the blind, the retarded, and the handicapped.

Timberlake, Bobbi. "The New Life Center." *American Journal of Nursing* 75 (September 1975), pp. 1456–1461.

Discussion of a center designed for couples who wish to become actively involved in decision-making related to childbirth. A description of classes that encourage participation in self-care is given.

Legal/Ethical Issues

Barchilon, J. *Malpractice and You.* New York: Ace Books, 1975, 304 pp.

Part One concerns such topics as what to expect from the medical profession; how to evaluate your doctor; and how to pick a good doctor. Additionally, information on what to do if you feel you are a victim of malpractice is presented in detail. Definitions of common legal and medical jargon are easily understood. Part Two consists of selected case histories. These illustrate various aspects of medical malpractice. Functional guides for common disorders of organ systems, common diagnostic measures for the organ systems, and a glossary of common terms help the individual equip himself for a visit to the physician's office. The book serves as an excellent introduction for the individual to select and understand the legal-medical process.

Dorsen, Norman, ed. *The Rights of Americans.* New York: Random House, 1972, 704 pp.

This is an unique reference book for the United States citizen. Rights of the individual are presented as recognized by the local and supreme courts, including the right to control one's body and the rights of mental patients. Rights are outlined and their viability discussed.

Frankfort, Ellen. *Vaginal Politics.* New York: Bantam Books, Inc., 1973, 224 pp.

The author advocates awareness by women of abuses by the medical establishment. The basic premise is that when women are more aware of their rights as patients, they can better protect their own health.

Jaworski, Suzanne. *Consumer Participation in Health Services: A Curriculum.* Vol. II: *Sourcebook.* Washington, D.C.: The Institute for the Study of Health and Society, 1050 Potomac Street, N.W., 1972.

This volume is a collection of articles dealing with the issues of community control and consumer participation. The topics in the articles range from the issues of community control to consumer participation in neighborhood health centers, the discussion of some consumer issues to the consumer health arenas. In addition to the bibliographies after each article, each section has an extensive listing of other relevant sources.

Landau, N.J., and Rheingold, P.D. *The Environmental Handbook.* New York: Ballantine Books—Friends of the Earth, 1971, 496 pp.

As a handbook, the consumer will find useful information on what environmental issues or abuses can be acted upon, what are the appropriate methods of action under certain circumstances, and what "tools" should be used in litigation, class actions, and citizen suits. Of interest to self-care is the orientation of the book to the de-mystification of the legal process and how the ordinary citizen can become more effectively involved in the legal process in cases related to health.

National Analysts, Inc., NTIS. *A Study of Health Practices and Opinions.* Philadelphia: National Analysts, Inc., 1972, 343 pp.

This study explores the nexus of health beliefs and practices in the United States by means of a large national survey and area probability techniques. Subjects investigated include use of vitamin pills; health foods; weight reduction practices; use of laxatives; self-diagnosis and medication; treatment of arthritis, rheumatism, and cancer; use of health practitioners; hearing aids and medication; aids to quit smoking; and general health attitudes and opinions. There is a clear value bias based on the supremacy of the medical model. Thus the stated purpose of the study "to investigate 'fallacious or questionable' health beliefs and practices and 'susceptibility' to them leads to such tautological action implications as the problem of 'rampant empiricism'—the irrational trial and error folk practices and psychosomatic suggestibility of the laity." Data analysis is weakened by shifting denominators and percentages of percentages.

U.S. Department of Health, Education, and Welfare. *Medical Malpractice: Report of the Secretary's Commission on Medical Malpractice* plus Appendix. Washington, D.C.: Department of Health, Education, and Welfare Publication No. (OS) 73–88, 1973, report 143 pp.; appendix 854 pp.

A massive report by a multidisciplinary panel of experts to the Secretary of HEW on the entire range of problems associated with malpractice. The report itself gives a brief summary of the findings with recommendations. The appendix provides detailed data about medical, legal, insurance, and consumer studies involving malpractice. A discussion of state laws about medical record disclosure is included.